# PALEO DIET FOR BEGINNERS

## Complete Guide for Rapid And Lasting Healthy Weight Loss

**Written by Mark Sell**

I0421930

# Table of Contents

## PREFACE

This book provides you the required knowledge, data and recipes to know the basics of Paleo-style and the way it will essentially remodel your life if you adopt this lifestyle. This book provides you with one in every of the foremost healthiest Paleo diet plans and following these diets can assist you to attain a lean physique and an overall healthy body and mind.

You will have additional energy throughout the day and can get much better sleep at nighttime, your skin and hair also will show a distinction in general health. This diet is additionally very straightforward to follow as you'd simply have to be compelled to eat lean meats, recent vegetables, and ocean foods. This book can show you the way to avoid ingestion modern-day foods that are extremely processed and contain colossal amounts of sugars and others have a high salt content. it'll walk you through the processes of a way to avoid sugary foods and the way to tackle the matter of sugar cravings with the assistance of paleo sugars.

Nowadays it's not regarding what quantity you're eating however in fact what you're eating and every one of those affects your health and fitness. during this present time of science and technological analysis, scientists have proved through various studies that consuming whole grains, dairy farm merchandise, and different processed foods lead to several diseases that embody polygenic disorder, heart diseases, obesity, cancer, and blood pressure.

But upon more reading, you will get to know how superb Paleo diet is and the way you'll be able to incorporate it in your life to avoid all of those diseases and live a healthy life. This book can create your intake easy and assist you to melt off fat and win the lifestyle that you just desired for a long time and restore your vigor and guarantee you an extended and healthy life.

# CHAPTER 1

## INTRODUCTION:

The Paleo diet is the healthiest plant in the world, requiring no starvation, and no horrendous, continuous exercise. It looks to how our ancestors ate, all those thousands of years before, when things like diabetes, obesity, and heart disease did NOT rule the earth as they do today. And, with that past diet plan, we discover a healthier way to lose weight, to prevent diseases, and to ward off serious mental issues, like depression and anxiety.

What our prehistoric ancestors ate are a few things that we won't be able to specifically verify. None people lived throughout those times and thus, it might be arduous to pinpoint specifically what they ate them. We cannot probably return in time, will we? At most, we can just build an informed however reliable guess supported no matter info we've got uncovered from the past. Supported various analysis studies, the kind of food prehistoric individuals ate were, for the most part, restricted to what was out there in their geographic locations throughout any given time. What they're are often deduced through meticulous scientific studies and advanced laboratory analysis of the prehistoric bones and dentures of Paleolithic individuals. Results from such studies served as a basis for our assumptions of what constitutes the primal diet.

We can conjointly build plausible assumptions on what constitutes the primal diet through sheer logical reasoning. By learning the kind of food we've got these days that couldn't probably have existed throughout the Paleolithic era, we must always additional or less be able to verify what style of food prehistoric individuals ever consumed through the method of elimination. By hanging out modern foodstuff that couldn't have probably existed throughout the stone-age era from our food list, we will be able to set out with a plan on what our ancestors ate.

For example:

they had no dairy farm product then as animals weren't however domesticated. it might completely be not possible and even too risky to take advantage of wild cows (if they already existed) or alternative fresh wild animals.

Agriculture wasn't existent then and thus Paleolithic individuals hardly had cereal grains. no matter grains they'll have had may are gathered from plants that grew wild within the fields that ought to be in for the most part restricted quantities.

They never salt-cured their food since they didn't have salt too at that point. There's no documentary proof existing these days that shows stone-age individuals mined salt throughout their era. the sole doable issue they might have done then was to dip their food in saltwater.

Sugar wasn't however out there too at that point solely usable sweetener they would have used is wild honey that we can assume was also arduous to seek out at that time.

Lean meat from wild animals was their common menu which suggests their diet had higher protein content compared to today's diets.

Their consumption of proteins is additionally low however wealthy in fiber compared to trendy diets as their carbohydrate supply come back from wild fruits and plants existing at that point most of that are non-starchy and thus have lower carbohydrate content.

They didn't have trans-fats like what we tend to typically get from processed foodstuff these days. What they had were omega3 fats, unsaturated fats and healthy monounsaturated fats from lean meat, fish, and food.

The Paleo diet offers an essential weight loss and healthy lifestyle plan. The diet plan works with the way your body has evolutionarily evolved to give you the food you naturally crave the food that will help you age well, live well, and drop pounds from your waistline.

The Paleo diet may be a diet not like any other diet out there as a result of the Paleo Diet isn't a diet!! Yeah, you heard that right. I hate the thought of a diet, and that I have a hidden suspicion that you simply do similarly. The Paleo Diet may be a fashion and once you see the light or during this case, feel the light, you may simply surrender all those unhealthy foods permanently. I'll show you the manner and hold your hand through this journey. Read through the book, try it, see how you feel, and evaluate your daily life and make adjustments accordingly. Every one of us is different and we all respond to foods and diets differently - Bottom line... give it a shot and see how you feel, because, at the end of the day, that's the only real science you need. Our diet and health should never be a constant thought in our minds. We eat to survive, and food is fuel for the body. Back in the days of our ancient ancestors, they didn't think about calories and fat content. The word "carbs" never came into their conversations. And yet they lived an extremely healthy and fit lifestyle and were able to have the energy necessary to hunt and gather food every day. Why is this the case? Why do you have to think so much about your daily caloric intake? It isn't about that. I want you to get 'counting calories' out of your mind right now. Once you fully grasp the idea of the Paleo lifestyle, you'll begin to see that this way of life has far more benefits than the typical American diet has to offer.

# CHAPTER 2

## The Paleo Diet versus the twenty-first Century Western Diet

What our prehistoric ancestors had been natural, unprocessed food that they forage or hunted inside their immediate geographic region. the trendy urban diet, on the opposite hand, is usually processed foodstuff dominated by sweetener and cereals and synthetically made ingredients. The comparison is a toss-up between what's natural and what is artificial. as to which one is best, we have to shall shall shall leave this up to your judgment.

But what has been construed because the Paleo diet truly has 2 to 3 times more fiber than the standard average Western diet. it has twice more unsaturated fats and monounsaturated fats and 4 times more Omega-three fats. A lot of important issue with this primal diet is that it's a half-hour to four-hundredth less saturated fats than the trendy urban diet. Its protein content is 2 to 3 times over the typical modern urban diet.

Since the Paleo diet contains moderate amounts of helpful fats and carbohydrates with low glycemic indexes and a load of useful phytochemicals, it's the proper diet to stop weight gain and avoid cardiac diseases. On the opposite hand, there are voluminous proofs that link the trendy urban diet to a high incidence of pandemic cardiac diseases and fatness nowadays. The monounsaturated fat content of the Paleo Diet comes principally from nuts and has been tested to guard us against cardiac diseases in a minimum of six clinical studies. The omega-three fat content is additionally higher within the primal diet than in the meat from today's domesticated animals since they're grain or corn-fed and not fed with polyunsaturated fatty acid-rich grass. Omega-three fat conjointly has cardio protecting properties. The saccharide content of the primal diet has a lower glycemic index than the carbs from modern diets since they primarily return from non-starchy fruits and vegetables. it's simply that the human body remains genetically tailored to the primal diet. whereas it's not possible to duplicate the diet specifically because it existed throughout the prehistoric era, it will serve as the rule of thumb to design effective diet interventions to guard man from the incidence of cardio diseases.

## The advantages and Disadvantages of the Paleo Diet

Since the Paleo diet gained prominence, it attracted advocates additionally as detractors. Naturally, the advocates can solely sing praises and heap accolades for this new dietary plan. On the opposite hand, its detractors are going to be fast to illustrate perceived flaws in its logic. For your sake, we are enumerating here all the arguments for and against the Paleo conception coming back from each side. we will leave the ultimate decision to your higher judgment.

The advantages of Paleo diet advocates proclaim that the diet provides a bunch of great health advantages among that are:

1. The Paleo diet protects against weight gain. Since the diet prescribes solely non-starchy fruits and vegetables as its main supply of carbohydrates and not from grains and sugar that have high glycemic indexes, the hypoglycemic agent levels within the blood are down so preventing carbohydrates from being born-again and kept as fat. It truly results in important weight loss within the long run.

2. Despite having high levels of saturated fats, the Paleo diet has been shown to boost blood lipid profiles. It will increase the positive sterol (HDL) levels whereas decreasing the TG or triglycerides so, effectively shielding the heart from coronary artery disease and stroke. It conjointly has been shown to convert less dense unhealthy sterol (LPL) into high-density smart cholesterol (HDL).

3. The Paleo diet is protein-free since it leaves out wheat and different cereals from wherefrom gluten are formed. It enhances digestion since the food intake is restricted to the kind of food the physical body has been acquainted with for many years.

4. The Paleo diet eliminates glucose spikes and maintains stable energy levels within the body. You typically won't get afternoon fatigues as what happens typically once you eat loads of cereals and sugar throughout the day.

5. It prevents bloating and promotes well being since there's a lot of fiber intake within the saltless diet. All of the food and beverages within the Paleo diet are organic. folks on the Paleo diet feel energetic, sleep finer, and aren't vulnerable to depression.

### The disadvantages

Critics of the Paleo diet haven't wasted time to post their criticisms. Among the various objections, they need thus far printed are the following:

1. The Paleo diet is simply too tough for the easy person to follow because it entails an amazing amendment in one's fashion. it'd take herculean efforts to visualize it through to success. With such a large

amount of food restrictions, it'll need changes not solely in your consumption habits however in buying food things since you would like to pick only organic food product and meat from farm animal that has been raised and grass-fed in pasture lands. it'll entail taking a better cross-check food labels to create positive they contain solely natural and organic ingredients.

2. The shift to a Paleo fashion is also dearer than usual. The fruits and vegetables ought to be organically mature and this positively can cost you higher than the regular fruits and vegetables sold-out anyplace. The meat should be from a eutherian mammal that has been grass-fed or fed with corn or grains. Paleo detractors also claim that the Paleo food list includes foodstuff that isn't solely less in supply however also is costlier.

3. Critics of the Paleo diet feels that by going out grains and cereals, the diet is in result depriving the body of abundant required fiber intake and carbohydrates. They think about the Paleo as an unbalanced diet. They conjointly feel it's absurd to use modern foodstuff to structure man's original ancient diet. They believe that Paleo advocates would have a problem to remain on the diet since critics believe that because it's arduous to find strictly organic and natural food sources. They predict that Paleo advocates are about to be discouraged and are seemingly going to abandon the diet shortly once they have tried it.

4. There's but, a typical ground among the advocates and also the critics of the diet. each party doesn't question the very fact that man ought to eat foods as natural and as contemporary as doable. this can be truly the terrible essence of the Paleo fashion and it seems that the higher criticisms are additionally like excuses to not adopt the diet than reasons to invalidate the effectualness of the diet.

**CHAPTER 3**

**Correcting the Misconceptions regarding the Paleo Diet**

Contrary to what the critics say, the Paleo diet is that the best and also the simplest diet to follow compared to different dietary regimens. It needs no calorie count. It simply desires a good resolve to stay to regular organic food intake and to avoid processed foodstuff and artificial ingredients. it's the healthiest too. Dieters are merely keen on creating excuses after they can't resist the urge of reversion to their recent consumption habits and succumb to the urges of their old cravings for things sweet. allow us to try and analyze the various misconceptions regarding the Paleo diet to raised appreciate its advantages.

**What is the Paleo diet?**

The Paleo Diet is largely a dietary idea supported on the assumption that by consuming in the like manner our stone-age ancestors did and limiting our food intake to the sort of food out there to the 2.5 million years agone, we'll become more fit, meaner, and healthier. it's over simply a bunch of well-concocted recipes. it's a full fashion that conjointly involves consuming modern food which is comparable to the food they ate and in the most state of nature attainable.

The Paleo diet isn't without any scientific basis. it's backed by historical proof, pure logic, and innumerable studies. a similar kind of transformative logic is applied to essential manner habits like sleep and exercise.

**What is the underlying logic behind the Paleo diet?**

The underlying logic upon that the Paleo Diet hinges based mostly on the assumption that the genetic composition of recent man has been programmed towards the diet man has been consuming since the time of our stone-age forefathers and it's not evolved a lot of since then. For over 2.5 million years, man has had a constant natural diet consisting of untamed plants and animals such a lot so that human genetics is believed to be already programmed towards this sort of diet and therefore the agricultural and technological revolution within the last 10,000 years has hardly affected it. this can be the transformative logic on that the Paleo Diet is predicated. there's proof that our ancestors were utterly healthy as they will be and are freed from the diseases Homo sapiens suffer from nowadays. Our genes additionally as our physiology evolved from an extended process of natural decisions that created a modern human being more suited to eat the food that their genes have evolved with for various years.

## How is that the Paleo diet different from alternative diets?

First of all, the Paleo diet isn't a reducing diet. it's property over the long run and promotes overall health and longevity. not like alternative diets, it's not targeted on achieving simply one, a specific goal like losing weight, enhancing performance in an athletic contest or just being an area of an illness management program. not like those diets, the Paleo diet promotes the health, well being, competitive performance and therefore the ideal weight of people by making hormonal balance within the body.

## What is allowed and what's not allowed within the Paleo Diet?

The Paleo diet encourages the consumption of food high in useful fats significantly those from animal sources, high in animal supermolecule, and moderate intake of natural carbohydrates returning from fruits and vegetables, nuts and seeds. The useful fats ought to embody saturated fats from oil, duck fat, lard, tallow, and butter in conjunction with monounsaturated fats from avocados and vegetable oil.

## Why must you get on this diet?

This is an easy, straightforward and simple to follow a diet that needs none of the cumbersome calorie numeration typical of different diets. it's the first diet humans are programmed to eat. Following this diet provides you a bevy of advantages that's unmatched by different diets. the advantages embody weight loss, muscle gain, higher digestion, stronger system, slowed aging, a lot of energy, quality sleep, less stress, better skin, and stronger teeth and bones among several different things. the most effective half is it protects you from several of the diseases of wealthiness that has infested modern humans for the last two hundred years like cardiovascular disease, diabetes, Crohn's unwellness.

## What would be a typical Paleo daily diet?

You can begin your typical Paleo day with a straightforward breakfast of 2 eggs cooked in butter with almond flour muffins and a few slices of bacon. For lunch, you'll be able to have Paleo chicken fajitas or Paleo salad summer wrap rolled in a leaf of romaine lettuce. they're simple to make. For specific preparation, directions see our Paleo lunch recipes. An afternoon snack will be one or two of macadamia nuts or almonds that ever you favor otherwise you can prepare a bowl of berries mixed with some coconut milk. Dinner will be a straightforward dish of cooked asparagus and mushrooms fancy with minced contemporary rosemary springs.

## Are bacon and eggs healthy?

Eggs from free travel chickens feeding on natural diets of plants and insects and bacon from grass-fed, pasture born and raised placental ought to be free from antibiotics, artificial food supplements, and growth-boosting hormones. they're natural and organic and are so healthy. Organic egg yolks and bacon contain generous quantities of useful polyunsaturated fatty acid fat and smart cholesterin. each contains healthy saturated fat that is crucial for the economical operation of just about each cell in our body. Besides, saturated fats ought to even be our main supply of calories over the carbohydrates. A modest quantity of common salt within the bacon or egg is healthy. As for those that dislike the chemical group in bacon, there are nitrate-free kinds of bacon on the market in the supermarkets. Nitrates are present compounds and may not be a priority. they will be found in a lot of higher doses in much all vegetables. "Cavemen eat this sort of diet as a result of which they are more physically active" Nothing will be clear of the reality that this story floated around by detractors of the Paleo diet. whereas the prehistoric cave dweller was indeed a lot more physically active than the common modern human these days, he didn't eat on purpose as a result of the physical activities he engaged in. He ate to survive and whenever he may, he would conjointly realize a while to relax, take a nap, and have a decent night's sleep. The principle behind the caveman's diet is easy enough for individuals to grasp and appreciate. once you are extremely active and have interaction frequently in daily exercises, you burn a lot of-of the sugar reserves referred to as glycogens that are stored in your muscles and liver. they have to get replaced otherwise you won't have a similar level of energy for the same activity subsequent time around. To remedy this and restore your strength and stamina you wish a lot of macromolecule intake. In different words, you'll be able to afford to possess a lot of macromolecule intake than the common person as a result of your physically active style. Corollary to the present, an individual who hardly exercises and spends most of his waking hours behind a table or on a couch look TV should eat fewer macromolecules otherwise any excess carbohydrate intake are going to be regenerate and keep as fat leading to weight gain and ultimately fatness that threatens to shorten your existence on earth.

## Why is sugar prohibited within the Paleo Diet once it's natural?

Sure enough, sugar is usually a present substance. we discover it in virtually everything nature produces. However, once it's refined into focused granules or powder and used intrinsically like we tend to do these days it becomes poison to the physical structure. it's now not in its natural diluted type. Continuous consumption of sugar will cause spikes in blood glucose levels which can induce strokes or result in other health issues like polygenic disorder. Fruits are the foremost ideal sources of sugar and carbohydrates as a result of the absorption of sugar from the fruits we tend to eat is tempered and over-involved by its high fiber content. Besides, the vitamins, phytonutrients, and antioxidants within the fruit stop injury to the cells once the sugar is oxidized at the cellular level. They additionally repair no matter damage could have already been done to the cells as a result of the reaction of sugar. we've full-grown accustomed to obtaining our sugar fix by adding teaspoon jam-packed with sugar to the food we tend to eat and also the beverages we drink while not realizing we are inflicting heavy injury to our bodies. it's time we tend to get our sugar fix from a lot of natural sources like fruits. it's safer and healthier that means.

## Cavemen died young, therefore why do we tend to adopt their diet?

Again, this can be another one in each of the numerous myths being floated around by detractors to discredit the Paleo diet. the reality is there's proof that shows that our Paleolithic ancestors lived longer than what the majority thought. several of them who died young, died within the hands of different predators or by being gored by their prey whereas on a pursuit. Others died of starvation or accidents, however, hardly any of them died of natural cause or health problems. the sole reason why modern humans live longer these days is as a result of he has access to advanced medical aid and technology and not as a result of his diet. Infectious diseases will currently be for the most part contained and neutralized. while not trendy medical facilities individuals these days would die early. And, on the contrary, there's mounting proof linking the fashionable urban diet to such life-threatening health conditions like cardiovascular disease, cancer, excretory organ and liver issues, diabetes, and different diseases of affluence.

## How am I able to keep Paleo notwithstanding I dine out often?

If you're on the Paleo diet, you must not have any worries if you've got to travel and get on the road for some time. Neither must you worry if you suddenly commit to treating yourself or your family or friends to dinner out of a whim. you'll be able to keep Paleo wherever ever you go. the sole hurdle would be you - however resolute you're in sticking to the Paleo style no matter you are doing, wherever ever you go, and whichever state of affairs you'll end up in. within the 1st place, there are Paleo friendly restaurants scattered everywhere the country and their variety is on the increase. You shouldn't have a problem finding one to eat in. it's not such a lot just like the previous days wherever you'd seldom realize restaurants that serve protein-free and strictly organic dishes. Today, protein-free and organic is the 'in' factor among restaurants from the high finish elegant restaurants to the regular sustenance chains and mall food retailers. These Paleo-friendly restaurants are germination like mushrooms everywhere in the country and several major cities all over the globe. There are even Paleo food trucks roaming around some cities serving strictly Paleo dishes on the enter street corners and parking tons. Before you continue a visitor before you eat with friends and family, build it a habit to see out that Paleo-friendly restaurants are settled in the area wherever you propose to travel. List down these restaurants before you permit the house for the trip or the planned dinner with friends or family. Don't live the house while not this list. you'll be able to do an internet search for Paleo-friendly buildings or check our restaurant list during this eBook. There could also be times you'll end up during a state of affairs wherever you get invited by friends to eat in a non-Paleo friendly building. Won't be back to raise the waiter if they need protein-free dishes. At a similar time feint an excuse why you wish your meal to be protein-free like having a heavy hypersensitivity reaction to grains and meals with traces of grain in them will be fatal to you. you'll be able to make sure they'll take this seriously as a result of if there's something building owners worry most it's having a client develop a health condition as a result of their food. Oh, and don't forget to inform them to not use oil in the preparation of your meal. Feint a similar 'allergy' excuse. follow your Paleo diet even once eating out with friends in restaurants or once you get invited for dinner in their homes. Don't desire the 'odd man out' once you refuse some food. However, once you refuse a number of the foods they serve you wish to elucidate why so that they won't feel slighted. simply make a case for that what you refused could do some injury to your health. you'll be able to take this chance to debate with them the Paleo diet and also the advantage of eating healthy. who knows? you'll nonetheless win them over to the Paleo style. And notwithstanding they don't convert to Paleo you'll be able to a minimum of making sure that subsequent time they invite you over they'll prepare one thing that's Paleo for you.

### Should I be going back to a traditional diet when I reach my targeted weight?

Many people who press on a diet desires to slenderize most so that they assume that each one forms of special diet Paleo included is merely for losing weight. To them, something with the word 'diet' has become synonymous with weight loss. However, the Paleo diet is quite simply a weight loss formula. it's not one thing you ought to discard when achieving your ideal weight. it's instead a formula for a healthy manner that you would have to embrace for the remainder of your life if you would like a disease-free, healthier body and an extended lifespan. Besides, it makes no sense to travel back to a diet that within the initial place is that the main reason for your being overweight. Of course, you absolve to do as you want together with going back to your recent consumption habits and exposing yourself all over again to heart diseases, diabetes, and different modern-day afflictions that hounds man these days. It's your choice however make it sensible. If you have got reached your ideal weight on the Paleo diet it suggests that it's effective and there's a lot of reason currently to remain on with it. however please note that weight loss is simply a part of the helpful effects of this diet. it'll heal the harm done by a trendy urban diet has done to your gut and still balance the hormones in your system. this may take it slow to realize which suggests you continue to keep doing Paleo even long after reaching your ideal weight. Anyway, if you keep Paleo for a few time you'll get accustomed to it and notice it not solely delicious however additionally fulfilling.

### Shouldn't we tend to eat meat the manner the cavemen did?

The ideal Paleo diet ought to embrace each raw and prepared meat. there's but a sub-category of Paleo adherents who believe that consumption solely raw Paleo meat is that the ideal diet. The decision it Raw Paleo. Their variety remains little, however, it's growing. On the opposite hand, the bulk of Paleo advocates value more highly to have their meat prepared. it might be incorrect to mention that cavemen invariably ate their meat raw. maybe they did before they found the way to begin starting fire. however once man learned the way to begin starting a fire he additionally learned to cook the food he ate. And there's overwhelming proof that dates for several years to prove he did. preparation makes meat a lot of eatables and absorbed by our systems. whereas preparation indeed destroys abundant of the meat's nutrients, it properly compensates for this by making prepared meat simply eatable and extremely absorbable. no matter nutrients are left within the prepared meat, they simply reach each a part of the body together with the brain, nourishing and dashing up their growth and development within the whole process. it's no surprise then why man's brain developed quicker than those of the remainder of the kingdom. Our brain is greater than those of the opposite animal species and this can be as a result of the learned to cook the food he ate that made the food easier to digest and also the nutrients promptly out there to be used by each cell within the physical body. It wouldn't be, however, to assume that our Paleo ancestors prepared their food as extensively as we tend to do these days. At the onset, they have to have tried experimenting with it and their diet must have been a mixture of prepared and meat. Certainly, there's space for meat within the modern Paleo diet. The optimum Paleo diet ought to be a mixture of raw and done. And if you don't have the abdomen for meat, you'll be able to at least cook it rare or medium-rare. Or, you'll be able to eat raw fish and home-cured dishes for a change in food.

## How much fat, proteins and carbs do I eat?

Unless you're an endurance athlete exercising in preparation for an athletic event, there's no enumeration of calories or activity of fat, protein, or sugar intake for your Paleo diet. And albeit you're an athlete there's no atomic number or quantitative relation of food intake that everybody should follow to achieve optimum results the Paleo diet. what proportion fat, protein, and carbohydrates an individual desire depends on his individual needs and private circumstance. just in case you haven't noticed, the dietary recommendations of every one among those promoting the diet differs slightly from each other. There are hardly any 2 recommendations that are precisely alike once it involves suggested dietary intake. this can be as a result of completely different people who have different physical build, health condition, personal preferences, and fitness objects. Some merely prefer to slenderize. Others are a lot of into rigid physical learning in readiness for future athletic competitions. There also are people who are into the Paleo diet as a part of a health maintenance program to cure reaction diseases. Naturally, the nutrient demand depends on individual needs which cannot be similar to those of the opposite people with completely different requirements or nutritionary needs. Certainly, the Paleo diet isn't any remedy or a cure resolution for people who would like to pursue a healthy manner or no matter their objectives perhaps. Paleo isn't sort of a 'one size fits all' form of a diet. And, the best approach to following the diet is to simply eat no matter is natural and organic together with tons of helpful animal fats. The safest combination ought to be high fat, low carbohydrates, and moderate supermolecule. But again, how high is 'high' and the way low is 'low' can depend upon individual desires and needs. There are extremely no rules written on a stone for individuals to follow. you will adopt a selected Paleo diet recommendation however you may have to be compelled to check that changes to suit your personal preference or style. however so long as what you eat is natural and organic and belongs to the Paleo food list, it'll still be Paleo. The Paleo diet for endurance contestants may be a completely different story particularly if the athlete is on to a rigorous coaching regime. in step with good shape coaches a contestant who ought to consume two hundred to three hundred calories from straightforward to digest sugar sources an hour before his scheduled exercise with another 200 to 300 calories each hour thenceforth for the length of his work out. He additionally needs to take another two hundred to three hundred calories within a half-hour when the exercise to assist the body to recover from the strenuous workout.

**Are supplements allowed?**

Doctors would unremarkably advocate supplements to persons with specific health conditions in line with severe victuals deficiencies otherwise they'd instead recommend a diet made within the deficient vitamins or minerals. The Paleo diet is already dense in vitamins and minerals that the body desires. Unless the deficiency is serious enough to want 'shock treatment supplements are whole extra. Besides, most supplements are synthetically created. Or, they'll return from organic extracts however they still contain artificial ingredients. they will do a lot of damage than good to your body within the long run. If you're on the Paleo diet there's no more need for supplements. it'll simply be a waste of your cash since the diet has all the nutrients you would like. All you would like to try and do is stick with the diet and let it heal your body naturally – while not supplements. provides it a decent time to figure your body and heal it from years of injury caused by the food you've been consuming. In time your gut can finally have the best secretion balance it has to operate expeditiously. If you're from a northern county or work inside most of the time likelihood is that you are vitamin d deficient. go out under the sun more typically and for extended periods. You'll get all the vitamin d you require from daylight. what's good is that it's free.

## Is there a settling period to the Paleo diet?

Weaning over to the Paleo diet from your recent diet might} would like may need an adjustment period of nearly three to four weeks. it's no joke to form a fast shift to a less carb diet once your body is so accustomed to being bombarded with high carb doses every day for several years. you will encounter some lightheadedness or feel lightsome most of the time. you will even be jittery and irritable. These are traditional bodily reactions if you begin taking under fifty grams of carbohydrates that is all that the Paleo diet can provide you with every single day. however, don't worry as a result of these withdrawal symptoms can presently glide by. And as you get accustomed to the diet more and more daily, you may begin to feel extremely energized. The Paleo diet features a detoxing result on your body. It starts to urge obviate the toxins that have accumulated in your muscles cells of these years. These toxins are discharged to the bloodstream and ultimately excreted out of your body by your system. you may be experiencing detoxing symptoms like lightheadedness or irritability throughout this stage however this can be solely temporary. you may solely feel such symptoms whereas the diet remains cleansing your body and subsequently you will feel energetic and active.

## How much concerned should I be regarding withdrawal symptoms?

You may undergo alkaloid withdrawal headaches or the alleged 'low carb flu' manifested in ways that like feeling weak, feeling tired, having headaches, or equally light-weight symptoms. you don't need need to not worry because they're going to disappear in a matter of a few days. simply stay resolute and follow the diet. everybody who switched over to the Paleo diet perpetually become to be grateful as a result of the discomfort they went through for a brief amount of time was nothing compared to the immeasurable advantages they gained from it.

## How long can it take before I begin feeling accustomed on a Paleo diet?

After fourteen to thirty days on the diet, the typical person ought to begin feeling the total useful effects of going Paleo. Of course, this might vary from person to person reckoning on how they strictly follow the diet. If you go strict Paleo right from day one you will undergo more intense however shorter detoxing syndromes. But, you'll feel far better from the fourteenth day and onwards.

**Aren't fish and food dangerous owing to high levels of mercury in them?**

Fish or any food for that matter that has high levels of mercury is unsafe to your health. this can be very true for industrially created farmed fish or those who are raised in fish pens or cages. However, the reality is fish caught wild from the ocean has less mercury content than the vegetables we tend to purchase from the market. Fish ought to be an integral part of the Paleo Diet as a result of it's the most effective supply of high levels of Omega three. that's why in the coming time you purchase fish you must check the labels to know for certain it's not farmed fish however fish caught from the ocean. the higher possibility is to shop for fish from the fisherman's wharf if you reside close to one.

**Is the Paleo diet a mere fashionable diet?**

The Paleo diet is over-programmed food intake. it's a complete style that revolves around uptake solely natural and organic foodstuff. It can't be a fashion since this type of diet has been existing for innumerable years. it's property for a lifespan and not one thing individuals will simply lose interest as time goes by.

**Isn't this similar to Atkins?**

Many people erroneously suppose, therefore. On the onset, they sometimes do look similar however if you cross-check them closely you'll discover that there are vital variations between the 2 that sets them apart. For one factor, the Paleo diet permits you to eat as several contemporary fruits as you wish – no restrictions whereas Atkins solely allows controlled servings and not all fresh fruits are allowed. however, the foremost vital distinction between the 2 is that the proven fact that the Atkins diet permits the consumption of heaps of processed meats and saturated fats. The Paleo diet, on the opposite hand, bans all processed meats and puts stress on animal macromolecule and useful fats from grass-fed, free from farm animals solely.

## Can the Paleo Diet assist you to lose weight?

The simple answer is affirmative. Weight loss is, however, a positive residual result of the Paleo diet. Its real price is keeping you healthy, fit, and feeling such a lot better for the long-term. don't expect it to be a fast fix for weight gain. you'll slim down o.k. however, it won't be very dramatic. Rather, it'll be a gradual method that creates it extremely manageable and long term and a lot of permanent. With the Paleo diet, the body is instructed to use fat for energy and limit its dependence on carbohydrates for energy. within the method, there'll hardly be any excess fat to behold on and no matter fat is there will be regenerate into energy to power cell functions. you furthermore may get to avoid high supermolecule intake which may cause spikes in glucose levels. rock bottom line is that the majority of individuals who adopted the Paleo diet achieved vital weight loss once being within the diet for a considerable time. the great news is it forever corrects the body's dependence on carbohydrates and you'd be able to maintain your ideal weight with hardly any effort.

## What am I able to get from following the Paleo Diet?

Weight loss is one among a lot of vital edges you'll gain from following the diet. There are heaps of other different edges it provides like progressing to sleep far better at night, improved skin complexion, improved sex drive (if you would like to think about it significant), improved digestion, clearer mind, and inflated energy. The Paleo diet heals your body back to its original condition very like overhauling an automotive and repairing broken components. It will cure such diseases as Crohn's disease and alternative response diseases.

## Won't you get bored consuming virtually identical foods each day?

Theoretically, the solution would be affirmative you will get bored. The Paleo diet doesn't have an in-depth line of luxurious recipes as what you have got been accustomed for years and should taste otherwise with sugar and salt deliberately disregarded. however, if you think about the fact that our body appearance for selection solely as a result of it's not obtaining the best nutrition from the food you eat then you'll better appreciate and perceive why Paleo converts are sticking out to the diet permanently. Your decisions of food on the Paleo diet are also restricted however they offer you the best nutrition that ultimately curves your cravings for selection. Besides, it's not true that the Paleo lacks selection. The Paleo recipes enclosed during this book are simply some of the numerous Paleo dishes you'll notice around. and that they are by no means that less luxurious. individuals tend to consider the Paleo diet as another one among those bland and tasteless slimming diets. Nothing will be clear of the reality and therefore the thousands of recipes you'll discover online is proof of this. you'll have a range of healthy foods while not venturing out of the Paleo tips. whereas several prefer to follow an easy diet, you'll elect to possess a selection in your Paleo meals and an easy online search can assist you to do this with ease.

## Why do I need to avoid adding salt to my food?

Intake of salt additionally as grains, legumes, and cheese creates an extremely acidic setting in our bodies and puts tremendous stress on our kidneys. As a reaction response, the body is forced to trigger the calcium reserves in our bones to neutralize the acidity and restore balance all over again. the total result of this, however, ends up in chronic diseases like pathology.

## Grains have fibers, minerals, and vitamins, therefore, why ought to I take it out from my diet?

The little identified truth regarding whole grains is that they contain an indigestible substance referred to as phytate that stores energy and therefore the part phosphorous within the grain. Phytate is that the salt sort of phytic acid that binds the metallic element, iron, zinc, and calcium in our intestines and effectively leading them out of our bodies preventing them from being absorbed by our system. Mammals {including|as we tend toll as|together with} humans cannot digest phytate, as a result, we don't have the catalyst phytase. without that, it can't be digestible or absorbed leaving it to wreck mayhem by obstructing the much-needed nutrients we mentioned on top of from being absorbed by the body. This in result makes grains anti-nutrients. we tend to do need fiber in our diet fruits and vegetables will give the fibers we'd like. Fruits and vegetables are healthier sources of fibers than grain that do a lot of injury than benefit to our bodies. in contrast to the fibers found in grains, the fiber in fruits and vegetables is very soluble and is well assimilated into our system while not doing injury to the walls of the intestines that grain fibers notoriously do. On top of all that, fruits and vegetables contain a lot of B vitamins and folacin than grain. It won't add up to continue eating grain that has fewer nutrients and does a lot of injury to our system once we will get more nutrients from healthy sources like fruits and vegetables without having to risk damaging to our intestines.

## Can a vegetarian get on Paleo Diet at the same time?

The simple answer to this question is no. they need to settle on between the 2 as a result of the basic distinction that prevents them from a combination like water and oil. as an example, most vegetarians rely heavily on the utilization of grains and legumes like beans, peas, as their main supply of carbohydrates for his or her daily calorie necessities. As you well grasp by now grains and legumes don't seem to be allowed within the Paleo diet. they're anti-nutrients and cause chronic inflammation of the intestines a condition known as leaky gut that may be a precursor to several problems such as heart diseases also as cancer. Besides that, a strict feeder diet deprives the body of the much-needed nutrients, vitamins, and minerals that are unremarkably found packed in animal food sources. The feeder diet specifically ends up in deficiencies in vitamins D, B6, and B12 and essential minerals like iron, zinc, and iodine and useful nutrients like omega-three fatty acids and taurine.

## Is the paleo diet reaching to punch a hole in my pocket?

It is an incontrovertible fact that processed foods created in giant quantities are cheaper than organically grown fresh foods. There is not a  single doubt that the Paleo diet is going to be pricier than processed foods. However, if you're thinking that of the long run then let me tell you that it is going to free you from the travails of the fashionable urban diet and prevent from future medical expenses you're seeming to incur once you get afflicted with the numerous diseases as a result of prolonged consumption of processed food. In the end, you're probably going to be paying a lot of medical bills than the cash you saved by shopping for cheaper processed foods.

## Is it sensible to bring a Paleo pack lunch to work?

A packed lunch consisting of a vegetable dish flat-topped with grilled pigeon breast is simple to organize. Add an apple or a bag of nuts and pack some vegetables and you have got an ideal lunch to travel with. And if you don't have the time to organize a meal yourself you'll be able to attempt the prepacked Paleo meals that are currently obtainable from many online sources and in several selections. simply heat up it during a microwave at your office and you have got a hot, healthy lunch.

## Do I have to travel to a specialty food store to shop for my Paleo foodstuff?

Natural organic foods aren't solely obtainable in specialty outlets like monger Joe's. they will be found even in your neighborhood grocery store. you simply got to scan the labels rigorously. If you wish to make certain what you're obtaining is natural and organic then create it a habit to go to the farmer's market close to you. You'll get them contemporary there. For organic meat and poultry, the most effective manner is to induce them directly from certified producers. you'll be able to try this by a change of integrity any Community Supported Agriculture organization. I'm positive there's one close to you. Not solely are you able to make certain that you just can you get your meat and poultry from organically raised and grass-fed placental, however, you'd even be able to get contemporary and at remarkably cheaper costs.

## Is it an occasional carb, fad diet?

Critics say the Paleo Diet is simply another reducing diet that's low in carbohydrates and so unbalanced. Nothing may be clear of the reality that this unwarranted allegation. The Paleo diet isn't low in carbohydrates. Rather, its saccharide content has low glycemic indices since they are available from non-starchy fruits and vegetables. there's an enormous deal of distinction between having low macromolecule content and having carbohydrates that have low glycemic indexes. The Paleo diet encourages you to consume loads of fiber made fruits and vegetables that are its main sources of carbohydrates for energy. the trendy urban diet on the opposite hand depends on loads of sugar and cereals for energy that sadly causes spikes in glucose levels. It can't be reducing diet either as a result of man has been consuming this sort of diet even long before the appearance of agriculture. it's man's survival diet since it's been able to exist on this diet disease-free for many years.

## Is it tough to follow?

The most important issue regarding Paleo is that the incontrovertible fact that it entails no guesswork and needs no calorie count and constant observation.

it's a no-fuss dietary arrange that doesn't need you to perpetually make mathematical calculations or dine in the zone to make certain you're not overstepping through programmed dietary food intake.

# CHAPTER 4

## Blending your twenty-first CENTURY way to the Paleo Diet

One of the foremost tough things in incorporating changes to your 21 st Century way is in adapting the aforementioned changes to interchange established habits that don't change well to the new lifestyle. you wish to acknowledge which of them are often harmful to your efforts to attain healthiness and well being, therefore, you'll be able to do one thing to result in the changes. Here are a number of them:

If you're a tea or coffee lover and taking your morning coffee has become a daily ritual, you'll be able to plow ahead with it however you want to prune on sugar and cream. higher still take it strictly black low – no cream and sugar the least bit.

If your work keeps you busy all the time, you must survey the world around your office and establish the food shops that serve Paleo sort of foodstuff. never leave this to likelihood because if you do your set up can fail since you're probably to patronize non-Paleo food shops once hunger pangs get the higher of you before you'll be able to realize a building that's Paleo friendly.

If you slow down once to your cravings for the standard} food then you're probably to travel back to your old consumption habits and destroy your Paleo set up altogether.

If you're a cake and pastry enthusiast, you have got to give up your appetence. sweetener and farm merchandise don't have any place within the Paleo diet. you wish to work arduous to eliminate sweetener and flour from your way.

Remember that there's no area for compromise once you embrace the Paleo diet. Neither ought to there be the area for flexibility because it will destroy the diet utterly since you'll begin losing management over your consumption habits. If you're a fanatical social creature, you want to additionally prune on your nightlife or abandon it altogether. An active social life opens you to a lot of temptations which can probably force you to interrupt your Paleo diet. Don't eat food that uses oil, corn oil, soy oil or different oils made of grains and seeds. Restaurant food sometimes makes use of those oils and thus ought to even be avoided. Butter, lard and animal oil, unrefined copra oil, and vegetable oil ought to be used instead. don't be misled by claims that saturated fats are dangerous for your health. they're smart for your heart and your overall health. We shall be discussing this during a separate section.

Keep a tab on what you eat a day. begin your food diary and record not solely the food you eat but additionally, however you felt once every food intake. the info can assist you still adapt to the Paleo way a lot of simply. Our prehistoric ancestors never had an equivalent flood of food temptations you'll be featured with after you try and amendment over to the Paleo way. they'd no alternative attributable to their very existence relied on it. Besides, it had been the sole factor they'd so it wasn't onerous for them. The twenty-first Century man, on the opposite hand, includes a ton of tempting food selections to pick from every single day. He must, therefore, be ready to create concessions and may be willing to allow up to a number of his favorite food things if he's serious in adopting the healthy Paleo way.

## Adapting to the Paleo mode

### Eat just like a cave dweller

Adapting the Paleo mode to your own involves feeding the way the cavemen of prehistoric times did. No, it's not regarding moving within a cave and feeding there. it's not regarding scavenging or trying to find your food since you'll use modern food as a substitute. It is regarding consuming modern food that may not cause endocrine spikes. A spike in endocrine within the blood tricks our body to store energy as fat leading to weight gain. It is quite unfortunate that the fashionable man's diet is loaded with sugar and refined cereals. many of us these days are therefore accustomed to taking cereals for breakfast, packed sandwiches for lunch, and completely different food preparations for dinner. They even usually supplement this with snacks in between meals consisting of fries, chips, and soda. They couldn't care less about whether or not or not the continued consumption of processed food made in sweetener and cereals can create them gain weight quickly, and over time it's going to even cause polygenic disease or within the worst-case situation to cancer. Another issue that took to modern-day man's current difficulty is his mistaken belief on what represents a healthy diet. folks are brainwashed to believe that consuming low-fat foods high in carbohydrates can facilitate keep the heart healthy furthermore as stop weight gain. This thought is the offender. it's not intaking less fat and lowering carb intake which can forestall endocrine spikes. You'll solely be starving the body of abundant required nutrients that approach. The primal diet corrects this thought with a diet that contains a lot of healthy fats and non-starchy fruits and vegetables instead. it's not regarding limiting fat intake. it's regarding avoiding the utilization of trans fat and harmful omega-6 fatty acid fats from soy oil or vegetable oil that modern humans are utilizing extensively in preparing their food every single day.

## Going Primal needs Resolve

One should have the correct mental attitude before adopting the Paleo mode. it's essential that one should be resolute to avoid reverting into your previous rotten ways. Primal living is over a diet or a physical exercise program it's a complete mode amendment.

You need to understand the importance of feeding and acquiring ways in which our body is optimally designed. And it needs one to be unwavering once he starts going primal. it'll mean abandoning several things you've fully grown comfy with. it'd be like turning yourself far away from what used to be your ease zone and recharging yourself with a brand new Paleo mode. you furthermore maybe a lot of physically active. One of the sick effects of progress is it had made man lazy and quite less physically active such a lot in contrast to our prehistoric ancestors who are perpetually on the move trying to find food or looking for ways in which to shield themselves from the weather. Modern human beings spend the foremost a part of his waking time sitting in a workplace or look tv reception. Every day he'd ride his automobile to figure. Weekends are holy to him because it is that the solely time during a week he sometimes comes to life late and not worry regarding being late for work. Modern human being has chosen to adopt a way of life that slowly erodes his muscular health and ends up in cardiovascular degeneration. He must break from the labor of his day to day routine by going out underneath the sun more than he does and doing physical exercises.

**CHAPTER 5**

**What you have to give Up To Be Paleo**

So far, you recognize that you simply have to be compelled to surrender sweetener and cereals furthermore as legumes to be Paleo. however, there is more stuff you have to be compelled to surrender once you embrace the Paleo mode. Sacrifices can have to be compelled to be made together with venturing out of what accustomed be your comfort zone and preceding several things you love and are familiar with having. Among the items you have got to give up are the following:

**1. Avoid junk food chains**

Fast food and most different processed food material are high in trans fat and omega-6 fatty acid fats that cause inflammation. If hamburger and fries became a part of your routine, it's time to shed the habit. Stop creating holidays as food events Christmas, Thanksgiving, Easter, Birthdays, Anniversaries, etc. have forever been a food event. we've been at home with celebrating such events by making ready luxurious meals. it'll be tough to interrupt tradition however this must be left behind for you to be Paleo. inside a food fest, you should recommend a trek to the park or something else.

**2. Walk more, Ride less**

Your feet are created for walking. attempt to walk as usually as you're able to and whenever time permits. Leave your automotive behind whenever you'll and walk instead. Don't take the elevators and use the steps. it's smart for your heart. no matter ways in which you'll incorporate walking or any physical exercises to your leisurely fashionable mode aiming to be|are} a welcome amendment and is unquestionably going to boost your health.

**3. Resist the urge**

It is extremely tough to eat otherwise from the remainder of your friends. you will feel alienated or odd and therefore the temptation to allow in and eat non-

Paleo food with them is just compelling. However, there aren't any if's and but's with the Paleo mode and would have to resist all the urges and instances of yet again splurging on an unhealthy diet. Think of your health within the next 10 years. Be robust in your resolve and you will even gain your friends' respect for your new mode.

## 4. Prepare yourself for the future

Never assume that Paleo could be a miracle answer to uncontrollable weight gain. If you expect to lose pounds night long you will find yourself unsuccessful. it's a way of life that you wish to embrace for the remainder of your life. The results might not be dramatic however they're going to certainly come. {they may|they'll|they can} not be immediate however positive results will come back and therefore the changes are permanent.

## 5. Don't take medicine to cure your symptoms

Throw all the medications within the house out of the window. If your doctor forever prescribes medicine for any symptom, it's best to contemplate trying to find another one. keep in mind that what ails man is usually connected to the type of food he takes and this is often one thing your doctor should take into account. If you are taking up the Paleo challenge, you may facilitate yourself get eliminate these symptoms. you only got to be firm and resolute in adopting this new model.

## 6. Stop being a creature of habit

If you accustomed to bring out the children to eat out in some fancy restaurant chain each weekend or cook for them pancakes once they come back from college, it's time to interrupt the routine and prepare a lot of natural, healthier meals now around.

## 7. provide no excuses

One of the common excuses individuals use to justify feeding food is a hectic operating schedule. Drop the reasons. it's time to create firm changes on your food decisions if you want to pursue your health and fitness goals seriously.

## 8. head to the Farmers Market Instead

You may not be able to avoid getting to the grocery store for your house desires however take care to avoid the center section wherever most of the junk foods are. better still, you must visit the farmers' market close to you more than usual than the grocery store. They'll have many contemporary fruits and vegetables for you there.

## 9. Get a lot of Shine from the Sun

Don't avoid standing in the sun. it's healthy for you. Go outdoors as usually as you're able to. there's no more nutrient source for vitamin D than from sunshine.

## 10. reduce your dependence on fashionable gadgets

Instead of losing sleep browsing information superhighway or taking part in online games along with your iPad in bed, tuck it away and have a decent night's rest. rather than cardiopulmonary exercise or running around on specially designed shoes which will absorb shock, run barefoot. Weird because it could appear however it's extremely healthy for your body.

# CHAPTER 6

## What are the fundamentals of the Paleo diet?

The Paleo Diet is essentially a dietary construct engineered on the idea that by intake in the like manner our stone-age ancestors did and limiting our food intake to the kind of food on the market to them then, we are going to become healthy, leaner, and healthier. It's simply a bunch of well-concocted recipes. it's a full lifestyle that conjointly involves consuming the simple food in the most natural state. The Paleolithic era is what's unremarkably said because of the stone-age era. It marked that amount within the prehistoric human history wherever man started learning the way to craft varied tools out of stone. The word 'Paleolithic' comes from 2 Greek words that mean "Old age of the stone" or Stone Age for brief. it had been additionally the time once men discovered the way to build hearth and commenced change of state the food they ate. it had been an associate era that began regarding a pair of 6 million years past and all over simply 10,000 years past amount once agriculture and animal farming became notable to man.

It is, for the most part, believed that individuals throughout the stone-age era were primarily hunter-gatherers who survived by adornment along in tiny teams to hunt wild animals and gather edible wild plants for subsistence. These prehistoric men survived on minimally processed natural food for countless years and also the physical body was thought to own custom-made to that. The human ordering is believed to own evolved already programmed to urge its nutrients from natural sources when overwhelming identical minimally processed food for countless years. The advent of agriculture and agriculture simply 10,000 years past has brought profound changes to the manner individuals ate and also the kind of food that they had. As man's information grew, they additionally learned alternative ways to supply and method food a lot of expeditiously. Food began to be processed in ever-increasing scale quickly commutation natural food sources with that man has been wont to for countless years. the commercial revolution that ensued within the same era.

To completely perceive how this lifestyle amendment goes to assist you within the long-term, it's essential that you just perceive the fundamental core elements of the foods you eat. Now, I promise that I'll create this as fascinating as possible, however, it's vital that you simply perceive these elements because this is often what's progressing to structure the core of your diet. We're progressing to set out with one amongst my favorite groups: proteins.

## Proteins

Proteins are one of the core sources of life, they are responsible for the growth of our nails, hairs, and muscles. They also act with a lot of other enzymes and hormones in our body and have been a great source of energy for humans since the start of human life on Earth. They are present meat, eggs, fish and some vegetables and the humans have been utilizing them from the start to support their growth. They are also responsible for making our muscles grow and giving us the strength to do work. There are two kinds of proteins namely top-shelf proteins and bottom shelf proteins and both of these have their benefits for the human body. In the Paleo, lifestyle Protein plays a vital role and hence they cannot be neglected. They will form the basis of your new paleo lifestyle.

## Carbohydrates

If you're an Olympic contestant, carbohydrates are a vital part of your diet. And if you're an athlete or muscle-builder, carbohydrates also can be a vital bit of your diet. the matter, however, is that society has outlined carbohydrates in such a way that provides them a foul name when in reality they're a vital a part of our diet - when utilized properly. That last bit is essential because carbohydrates will be used into 2 separate teams, quite like proteins. while not obtaining too technical on you, we've got monosaccharides and disaccharides. "Mono" merely means that one sugar and "di" simply means 2 sugars. this is often why we are progressing to focus on the carbohydrates that'll truly facilitate your body to improve energy levels and help your digestion at a similar time. We'll get into the various sorts of carbs in a bit.

## Insulin

One of the most important indicators of fat storage needs to do with the internal secretion we tend to call insulin. you'll have heard of the term 'insulin' thrown around before on TV or seen it on the net - and there's a decent reason for it. insulin is essential in controlling your glucose levels, your body fat, and conjointly deals with aging factors. to measure an extended and spirited life, we want to give in our best to keep our insulin levels on the low aspect by controlling the foods we tend to put in our body - specifically, carbohydrates that tend to spike insulin and cause your body to store fat. to grasp insulin, we've got to additionally inspect insulin's role in controlling our glucose levels. Insulin's primary role is to inform the nutrients you set into your body where to be kept. If you're perpetually golf stroke high saccharide meals and sugar-coated foods into your system, your insulin levels spike and your body tell itself to store that energy as fat. this is often why the Paleo style avoids such foods and permits your body to the method itself and regulates insulin levels with efficiency.

## GRAINS!

When you make the jump and choose to undertake Paleo or dive in fulltime, it's vital that you just perceive the one essential ingredient you would like to eliminate from your diet - Grains. Grains embody everything from Barley wheat, corn, oats, rice and so on. however as comfy as you're feeding these items, it's vital to understand that grains are way less nutrient than traditional vegetables, fruits, nuts, and proteins. Grains have a name for stimulating improper liver, thyroid, and duct gland responses in many folks which might, in turn, result in reduced immunity, fungal infections, skin issues, anxiety, depression, and weight gain. one amongst the issues with grains is that they inhibit the body from properly digesting them. This goes back to the means that they were evolved as a plant species with no defense reaction. Our bodies simply aren't adapted to digest these sorts of grains - period.

**When you compare grains calorie for-calorie to different natural foods**

such as lean meats, seafood, and veggies, you perceive that they're an away weaker form of calorie and not appropriate for sustained energy. And this suggests that you just can't eat stuff like quinoa. I do know plenty of individuals out there have found quinoa to be an alternate to whole-grains, however, those don't fly, as well. because they're within the same family as grains, they still have identical forms of side effects on the digestive system as a grain. the most important issue you've got to stress concerning is that the mayhem they make on your digestive system. they incline to cause what's referred to as malabsorption that, in turn, affects your health and well-being. Let's re-examine a couple of-of the problems associated with attempting to soak up grains in your diet:


1. For starters, grains tend to break the liner of the gut. once the gut is broken, your ability to soak up nutrients is greatly diminished. we want the healthy lining of our abdomen to soak up all the nutrients we need for our bodies. This includes all proteins, fats, carbs, vitamins, and minerals.

2. there's additionally the danger for the gall bladder to be broken. this may inhibit the production of digestive juice, which suggests we are going to not be ready to absorb essential nutrients like vitamins A, D, and K. If you can't absorb these vitamins, then you're going to have a problem absorbing essential nutrients that you just do would like.

3. Once your gut lining goes, it opens the door for pathology deficiencies and cancer. Not Good. The exocrine gland is particularly full of inflammation caused by grains passing through. this could cause carcinoma or inflammation of the exocrine gland.

4. Bottom line is... grains

aren't meant for the body and may cause digestive system issues, which can, in turn, result in additional serious issues like degenerative disorder, atrophic arthritis, lupus, vitiligo, narcolepsy, autism, and a range of different diseases. Now, I do know you'll be saying, "But, I don't have any of those diseases!" I do know, however you've got to grasp that over time, these are the problems that arise after we don't look out of our bodies and expeditiously fuel them with the proper nutrients and whole foods.

**Gluten**

Gluten comes from the Latin word for "glue" that is that the 1st clue that this ingredient shouldn't be placed into the bod. protein could be a form of supermolecule that's found in wheat, rye oats, and barley, and it's the ingredient that helps the dough rise and provides the food its bouncy consistency. we aren't reaching to dive deep into what protein is, however, I would like you to understand it isn't smart for any folks, and it's vital to eliminate it from your diet. I'm not reaching to beat around the bush... whether or not you would like to listen to it or not, grains aren't that healthy for you. I do know I same it! of these foods style smart. The bread, pasta, cookies, you name it – they're all extraordinarily delicious. however, you've got to see past your style buds for one second to induce to the important truth of the matter and to grasp what foods can truly help you live and not kill you. Let's dive into the anatomy of grain to comprehend it. All grains are comprised of 3 parts: reproductive structure, bran, and germ. If that sounds weird, simply bear with me for a second here. As I said, I'm supplying you with the nuts and bolts of the boring stuff so you'll understand the Paleo diet and have enough information to create a choice concerning whether or not it's the proper lifestyle for you. I feel everybody will have the benefit of eating Paleo, however, this is often ultimately one thing you've got to do for yourself and gauge however well you're feeling. Ok, back to grains:

**Bran**

Bran is that the outer covering of whole, unprocessed grain. It contains some vitamins, minerals, and a bunch of different proteins and anti-nutrients designed to forestall the predation or uptake of the grain.

**Endosperm**

The reproductive structure is starch with a touch little bit of protein. this is often the energy provider of a growing grain embryo.

**Germ**

The germ (sometimes cited as cereal germ) is that the portion of the grain that acts as its procreative system. In nature, the cereal grain is distributed by the wind, and once everything falls into place, the embryo begins the method of growth mistreatment the reproductive structure for energy. this is often the place where edible oil usually derives from.

**A Note concerning Oats**

I perceive that there are heaps of individuals out there who like to eat their morning oatmeal. however, I have some dangerous news… oatmeal contains many proteins kind of like protein. These proteins are laborious to digest, and so stay intact despite the simplest efforts of the digestive process to break them down. quite a bummer, right? Well, let me simply place it this way… attempt your best to travel with none form of grains for thirty days and see however you're feeling. I guarantee that you'll notice a significant distinction within the manner your digestive system, your energy levels, and your overall health and vitality work. I would like you to induce the term "whole grain" out of your head for the length of this experiment. this is often a term employed by the govt. to urge the US to assume that whole grains are a healthy substitute for natural foods.

**A Word concerning Beans And Dairy**

Several diets in today's diet world have incorporated the utilization of beans (or legumes) as a healthy substitute for carbohydrates and proteins at intervals your diet. Beans aren't essentially evil, however, they are doing results in similar issues as grains. Gut irritation, anti-nutrients, likewise as inflammation. I do eat black beans from time to time if I want I'm not obtaining enough carbs from my fruits and veggies.

## Fats

Fats appears to be one amongst the foremost confusing aspects of the Paleo diet these days - and permanently reason. Ever since the office got concerned about the food processor, we've been told that fat could be a dangerous issue. this could be the reason however we've got to think about fat as a new price to every one meal we tend to eat. the overall population doesn't have a tough time understanding that carbs aren't smart for you. however once it involves fat, we are within the dark most the time. The funny issue concerning fat is our bodies are created of heaps of it. This includes our organs, brain, nerves, and even generative hormones. however, to accurately perceive however fat helps the body, you've got to grasp the subtypes of fats. There are 3 sorts of fats: saturated, monounsaturated, and unsaturated. You don't need to perceive everything concerning the science behind it, however, it's smart to grasp the fundamentals thus you're not within the dark.

## Monounsaturated Fats

This type of fat is usually cited as monounsaturated fatty acid and is found in the main in foods like avocado, olive oil, and nuts (almonds, walnuts, etc.). however, this sort of fat is additionally found in grass-fed beef, which happens to be one amongst the staples of the Paleo diet. These fats are quite superb, as they incline to assist improve insulin sensitivity, improve hormone response, and reduce sterol levels.

## Polyunsaturated Fats

While monounsaturated fats are usually thought of as a healthier form of fat, unsaturated fatty acids are higher for you than saturated fatty acids. this is often as a result of being noted to scale back unhealthy cholesterol (LDL) and increase smart cholesterol (HDL). unsaturated fats additionally contain essential fatty acids like omega-3 and omega-6 fatty acid. These are fatty acids that the body wants, however, it cannot essentially turn out on its own. These sorts of fats also are vital because they send a symptom to your brain to allow you to apprehend after you are full. this may forestall bad eating habits and may additionally assist you to lose weight. The bottom line, unsaturated fats are vital.

**Cut The Trans Fats!**

Let's simply say that trans fats aren't the simplest issue for you. however, I'm positive you've detected others mention this. Trans fats are created once unsaturated fats from foods like corn and soybeans are exposed to heat. The resulting fats look kind of like saturated fats. they need a name for damaging the liver operation and destroying insulin sensitivity.

**The Omegas (Omega-3 and Omega-6)**

These sorts of fats are vital as they assist in dealing with inflammation within the body, and are famous to assist control numerous cancer components (typically in something that's associated with inflammation issues). omega-3 fatty acids are classified as an anti-inflammatory drug, whereas polyunsaturated fatty acid is classified as pro-inflammatory. The goal with our nutrition ought to be to even the ratio between these 2 Omegas. the general public is lacking in polyunsaturated fatty acid, which might be satisfied with foods like wild fish, grass-fed beef, and a few egg sources. polyunsaturated fatty acid also can be taken in supplement kind, however, attempt to minimize the utilization of supplements the maximum amount as attainable once attempting to stay to a Paleo diet.

List of polyunsaturated fatty acid Foods

You Should Be Eating:

•Wild salmon

•Anchovies

•Mackerel

•Herring

•Trout

- Omega-3 Eggs
- Grass-Fed Natural Beef
- An assortment of nuts and seeds (walnuts and linseed, for example)

# CHAPTER 7

## The Transformative Logic of the Paleo Diet

The underlying logic upon that the Paleo Diet is predicated on the idea that the genetic composition of recent man has been programmed towards the diet of our stone-age forefathers and it's not modified since. For quite 2.5 million years, man has had a similar natural diet consisting of untamed plants and animals such a lot that the shape has already become familiar with it. The human genetics is believed to be already programmed towards this sort of diet and also the agricultural and historic period within the last 10,000 years has not remodeled it. This can be the transformative logic on which the Paleo Diet relies.

The premise states that the biological science of recent man had scarcely modified through these years even once the arrival of modern agriculture and animal farming and despite the big scale modernization of food handling. They believe the 10,000 years covering the time once man initially learned in what way to cultivate plants and domesticate animals up to now when the trendy urban diet evolved wasn't enough to reprogram human genetics. Besides, modern humans started following the fashionable urban diet consisting mostly of processed food barely two hundred years past such that it'd be not possible for the body to entirely reprogram what took it 2.5 million years to program. Worst, the body is reacting negatively to the trendy urban diet as manifested through numerous chronic diseases that currently plague humans.

It was a gastroenterologist by the name of Walter L. Voegtlin who initially toyed with the construct of the stone-age diet someday within the mid-70's. Since then, a variety of books and tutorial journals are written regarding it. Together, they show that there's increasing proof to prove that a diet consisting of lean meat, fish, fruit, and vegetables just like the diet of our prehistoric ancestors will stop the alleged diseases of wealth trendy men are currently usually afflicted with.

The Paleo diet grew in quality and as its acceptance was simply obtaining a kickstart, some authors and scientists tried to introduce some modifications to the current construct confusing some advocates within the method. Others questioned the validity of its therefore known as transformative logic while not providing proof to negate the construct. Never-the-less, the Paleo diet still captured the imagination of a growing range of health and fitness advocates and it currently seems it's here to remain.

Followers of the Paleo Diet believe that to make sure health and well being, and stay free from diseases of richness, Homo sapiens must adapt to a diet that resembles the diet of his prehistoric ancestors. This transformative logic of the Paleo construct didn't sit well with some quarters. A variety of dieticians and anthropologists, particularly people who champion alternative modern-day dietary programs have questioned its validity claiming that an abundant of the Paleo construct is simply supported guesswork.

True enough, all of the health professionals who championed the Paleo Diet support like Walter L. Voegtlin and Dr. Lorain Cordain didn't live nonetheless throughout the Paleolithic era to be able to have a primary account of what the prehistoric individuals had for his or her meals. primarily, we will say that almost all of the contentions they wrote regarding were mere suppositions. However, in spite of however presumptive the Paleo construct is, it's not entirely unsupported.

The truth is the way of the Paleo assumptions were culled from well-documented studies and in-depth laboratory analyses that embody thorough analysis of the dental perform morphology of Hominin Fossil Records and Paleoenvironmental modeling among others. The principles are scientifically sound, the logic extremely affordable.

We don't seem to be but, about to take into a lot of bookish aspects of the primal diet. What we tend to are more fascinated by whether or not following the diet above can facilitate people to stay healthy and free from the direful diseases and diseases that are joined to the fashionable urban diet. For us, we will provide no higher proof than the varied up to date hunter-gatherer tribes still existing nowadays in various components of the world who still live on an identical primal diet. there's the Hazda Tribe of Tanzania, the Veddas of Sri Lanka, and also the Mbuti pygmies in Congo, the Guyana Indians of the Republic of Paraguay, the Eskimos of Alaska, the Aborigines of Australia, and also the East Coast yank Indians. The chronic diseases of affluence Homo sapiens are at risk of are much absent among these tribes. they're the proof positive of how primal diet is very important to keep the shape healthy and illness free. If you would like a lot of scientific basis showing the efficaciousness of the Paleo Diet, here's one incontrovertible proof for you which of them Paleo detractors attempt to merely ignore as a result of they can not contradict it.

Researchers from the University of American state San Francisco (UCSF) headed by Dr. Timothy White and Dr. Linda Frasseto did an actual check on a bunch of individuals who were all thought-about as unhealthy or have a disorder of some type. The subject was given a Paleo Diet consisting of lean meat, contemporary fruits, fish, nuts, and vegetables. after simply two weeks on this diet, the pressure level of everybody within the group went down dramatically, whereas steroid alcohol and glyceride levels born a median of thirty points – a feat that in line with Dr. Frasseto would have taken medicine like lipid-lowering medicine and alternative cholesterol-lowering medications six months to attain.

There are uncounted alternative stories of however the Paleo diet helped unwell people regain their health several of that were never printed. innumerable accounts of how the diet helped improve the physique and therefore the the} performance of skilled athletes also abound. The diet isn't a mere fad as the majority are created to believe by its detractors. it's a lifestyle. in truth it's well on its thanks to changing into the lifestyle of the longer term – the exact reason why proponents of alternative dietary regiments {try to|attempt to|try and} discredit its real price by tagging it as a non-civilized approach of uptake and living. sadly, they need however to contradict its effectiveness that several of its advocates would swear to even with their own lives.

# CHAPTER 8

## Your Paleo searching List

It would be too oversimplified to mention that the Paleo diet consists of lean meat from grass-fed, free-ranging placental and organically big fruits and vegetables. However, this might be imprecise for people that are making an attempt at the Paleo for the primary time, therefore, we need to prepare a Paleo shopping list to guide you on what to shop for the future time you shopping for food.

## Lean Meat

Your main supply of proteins ought to be from the lean meat of naturally raised animals. Being naturally raised means that they were grass-fed (not grain or corn-fed) and are endocrine and antibiotic-free. consistent with executive department standards, lean cuts of meat ought to contain solely a complete of five grams of fat, no quite a pair of grams of saturated fat, and solely ninety-five milligrams of cholesterin per 3.5 ounces of serving.

They should be cut off all visible fat and cartilage the maximum amount as doable. you'll be able to eat the maximum amount of those meats as you wish and for as long as you follow these preparation tips:

Make sure you drain off all the surplus fat. never deep-fry meat to keep else fat to the minimum. Instead, attempt cookery, baking, or preparation. If you'll sauté any of them try and use as very little else oil as doable. Limit consumption of animal organs to eighty-five grams a month.

## The following are the suggested lean meat sources and therefore the selection cuts:

Buffalo or bovid meat (any cut), Beef (flank cut, prime cut of meat, bottom or top round, eye of spherical, and alternative lean cuts, beef ought to be ninetieth lean), Chicken (skinless breast meat, additional lean ground chicken meat), Turkey (skinless white turkey meat and additional lean ground turkey meat), Duck, Goat (any cut), Pork (Bone-in rib chop, bone-in cut of meat roast, tenderloin, boneless high loin chop and roast, center loin, ground pork that's ninetieth lean), Lamb (arm, leg, and loin, shank, ground meat should be ninetieth lean), Eggs from non-poultry raised chickens, Animal organs from the afore listed animals like kidneys, bone marrow, liver, tongue, and sweet bread, Game meats like rabbit, wild boar, or cervid (any cut).

## FISH

The micronutrients found in fish are found to spice up brainpower and development. Fish ought to, therefore, be a part of your everyday Paleo diet meals whenever attainable. Fish and alternative food are glorious sources of macromolecule and Omega three. keep in mind tho' to forever select fish caught within the wild over farmed fish. Avoid canned fish too. in contrast to meat, the fattier fish are additional nutrient since they contain more useful fats and alternative micronutrients and Vitamins A, C, and E. The supplementary common wild-caught fish you may notice within the market are: Salmon

## TUNA

Other ocean foods include Shellfish like shrimp, crab, lobsters, clams, mussels, and scallops.

## FRUITS

There aren't any restrictions for fruits within the Paleo diet. you'll be able to eat any fruit that you like and consume the maximum amount as you want. However, if you're attempting to lose some pounds, it's best to limit the consumption of dates, mangoes, bananas, watermelon, and pineapple. they need the most sugar content and it's best to consume them sparsely. Dried fruits need to be avoided as they're jam-choked with sugar. Eat more avocados due to the reason that they contain a load of healthy fats.

## VEGETABLES

All nonstarchy vegetables just like the dark-leaved greens, pumpkins, herbs, and

seaweeds are allowed within the Paleo diet. Starchy tubers like potatoes and legumes

## NUTS AND SEEDS

Raw, unseasoned dried fruits and seeds are a part of Paleo snacks. The list includes cashews, almonds, pistachios, Brazil and pine nuts, pumpkin seeds, flower seeds, herb seeds, flaxseeds, and pumpkin seeds.

## OILS

Avoid utilizing oil, groundnut oil or oil for preparation. they're extremely refined oils and per se have higher concentrations of inflammation inflicting unsaturated polyunsaturated fatty acid fats than the inflammation-reducing omega-three fats. Use instead the following: Virgin copra oil for every type of preparation Avocado oil for sauce or for low heat cooking vegetable oil for any quite cooking and as a salad dressing too vegetable oil for seasoning and low heat cooking walnut oil for seasoning flaxseed oil not for cooking or seasoning except for direct intake as omega-three supplement. the utilization of those Paleo counseled oils can facilitate maintain the balance between the omega three and omega half dozen fatty acids in our body.

## Paleo Beverages

Soda and alternative bottled beverages are out of the list. This includes bottled or canned fruit juices that are ordinarily high in targeted sugar. Below are the counseled Paleo-friendly beverages that can be used but without adding any extra sweeteners.

## Coconut Water

Drink sugarless coconut milk and resultantly it'll have various health advantages like antioxidant properties, it's advantages against polygenic disease, it provides you higher viscus health, keeps you hydrated and prevents urinary organ stones.

## Coffee

Drink black coffee or espresso, however, don't drink any lattes or sweet coffees as they're going to drive you far from your paleo lifestyle.

## PALEO TREATS and SWEETS

The Paleo lifestyle isn't all that uninteresting and drab. there's an area for infrequent alcohol as long as you don't make it in one drinking session. you will conjointly take pleasure in dark chocolates to your heart's delight. they're smart for the heart. If you're trying to find sweetener, use raw honey which is sold at the farmers market instead.

## Making Sure Your Meat is Paleo

Ideally, Paleo meat should be from free-ranging live stocks and are grass-fed instead of corn or grain-fed. Not only are they better, however, but they're also conjointly healthier and a lot more delicious. those who have tasted free travel chicken would swear to the current reality. Meat from herd animals that touched freely on pasture lands, and pigs and chickens set free on the sector are more delicious and quite a lot more nourishing. The primary ever staple food of our prehistoric ancestors is meat from wild animals they were able to seek out.

Paleo is regarding reversing the ill-effects of an excessive industrial enterprise to our lives that have conjointly modified our consumption habits dramatically. It's regarding consuming a lot more natural and organic food just like the cavemen did countless years past and therefore the meat was one among their 1st staple foods. just like the meat of our ancestors, the meat meant for inclusion in Paleo diets should be from a pasture-raised farm animal. Please observe that there's a giant distinction between pasture finished farm animal and the ones that are entirely grass-fed throughout their existence. Most of the pasture finished cows spent the primary half their lives subsisting on grain-fed diets and were allowed solely to cast the pasture to kill grass only before they're sent to the butchery. they're not entirely freed from antibiotics and artificial food supplements.

Buy solely AGA certified grass-fed meat. AGA stands for the American Grassfed Association. American Grassfed Association meat merchandise certification is a time they were weaned up to the time they were harvested. The association was a guarantee that the merchandise came from farm animals fed solely with grass from the pastures and was founded in 2003 by organic livestock producers, veterinarians, and a grazing range management specialists to push the grass-fed business. they need producer-members in almost every state and their merchandise is sold-out in supermarkets similarly to numerous farmers markets inside the immediate vicinities of their farms. you must not have a problem finding American Grassfed Association certified meat merchandise within the country. you will even order meat merchandise online from a number of these producers. For additional info on American Grassfed Association producers. purchase game meat whenever and where ever attainable. the simplest meat that approximates the sort of meat ingested by our Paleo ancestors is game meat. This includes rabbit, deer, buffalo, ostrich, and swine thriving within the wild. they're not tough to get as there are brick and mortar outlets furthermore as on-line shops wherever you'll be able to purchase game meat. they probably will be priced more than the regular meat sold in supermarkets however they're a lot more delicious, similarly exotic and healthier. There are restaurants too that feature exotic game meats in their menus.

Don't obtain farmed fish and ocean food. Farmed fish are those that are farmed in massive scales like shrimps, tilapia, salmon, and milkfish. Farmed fish and food don't get to eat their natural food. they're given an organic from grains instead. Farmed fish have sometimes high mercury content. confirm the fish or food you purchase isn't farmed however caught from the ocean, lake, or ocean and not industrially farmed on an oversized scale. how would you know? Inquire! Ask the seller where the fish or ocean food came from.

Don't obtain chicken and alternative poultry merchandise that was raised on a commercial scale. the likelihood is that they're grain-fed. hunt for free-ranging chickens. Don't assume they're onerous to search out. you'll be able to even shop for organically adult, free-ranging chickens in supermarkets however your best bet would be the farmer's markets. There are online sources too and possibly, identical sources wherever you purchase your lean meat additionally carry free-ranging chickens available for sale.

## The Paleo Guide to selecting chicken

### The Free-range Chickens

The free-ranging chickens, on the opposite hand, are continuously loose to freely go outdoors. they're allowed to kill plants and insects. They feed freely on their scrounging for food in their natural environment and allowed to grow on its own with no growth-boosting hormones or nourishment supplements. they're conjointly organic.

### The Organic Chickens

The organic chickens are chickens raised in giant numbers in a very wide, contained and controlled the atmosphere wherever they're allowed to additionally kill insects and plants. they're given solely natural organic feeds like vegetables however sans grain-based industrial feeds. Their atmosphere is herbicide, fungicide, and chemical-free. they're conjointly not given antibiotics or growth-boosting hormones.

### Chicken's nutritionary advantages:

The chicken meat has low sterol and fats but it is abundant in supermolecule and loaded with vitamins and minerals like vitamin B complex that is known to spice up the beneficial cholesterol (HDL) in your body, vitamin B complex that helps convert carbohydrates into fuel, element that are best-known inhibitors, an element that is required by the body for correct cell functions. Chicken meat is additionally a decent supply of supermolecule. Here may be a note of concern for you. If you don't wish to induce traces of harmful chemicals further from pesticides, fungicides, herbicides, and artificial food supplements and business feeds, it'll do the best for you to remain organic and stick with the Paleo food list.

## The industrial Chickens

The business chickens are raised in giant scales in overcrowded poultries or cages often sprayed with pesticides, fungicides, and herbicides. they're fed with grain-based business feeds and their growth is increased with hormones and victuals supplements whereas their health is fortified with antibiotics to protect against pestilence and sickness.

## Paleo Extreme: consuming Raw Food

People usually asked if Paleo is the caveman's diet then shouldn't consuming raw food be an integral part of it. the fact is that the Paleo diet encourages the consumption of food in their most state of nature as attainable. feeding raw food is, therefore, an important part of it. however, it's not such a lot as a result of our Paleolithic ancestors ate food that means but primarily because it brings important nutritionary advantages that should not be unnoticed. For one issue, raw food is live food. other than being wealthy in nutrients, it conjointly contains natural life energy. change of state food diminishes this life energy and destroys the nutrients considerably rendering it nutritiously useless. Doesn't it build a lot of sense to place living food into your body than food that has been rendered lifeless by cooking?

If the conception of live food and life energy appear unlikely to you, then at least take into account this. The food contains natural enzymes that facilitate break down the nutrients and aid the digestion and absorption of food. change of state destroys abundant of those enzymes. Of course, the body will manufacture these enzymes to assist within the digestion and absorption of the prepared food we tend to eat. however, it makes the bodywork tougher to supply enzymes when the body takes in prepared food and therefore the body will solely do most. On the opposite hand, the consumption of raw food saves the body from the difficulty of manufacturing these enzymes.

Cooking food at a hundred and twenty degrees Fahrenheit or higher destroys all the natural enzymes and far of the nutrients in them. consuming prepared food with abundant of the enzymes destroyed because of the change of state at high-temperature forces the body to supply these enzymes so unnecessarily adding stress to that. Raw food diet already contains these enzymes then it saves the body from this extra stress. well-liked raw food diets taken by most raw food converts incorporates raw and unprocessed fruits and vegetables, cracked and seeds, eggs, tuna dish from fish, Carpaccio from meat, not pasteurized and non-homogenized milk, cheese, and yogurt.

Raw food enthusiasts can swear that consuming raw food is an exceptional energy booster. They profess that it offers them a moment of energy recharge. They conjointly claim they get to sleep deeper when consuming raw food, thus, they have fewer hours of sleep than is generally needed. consequently, they continuously come to life feeling choked with energy all the time.

These are their claims however a lot of concrete advantages that may be gained from a raw food diet in line with nutritionists include:

Significant weight loss - since it's primarily a coffee fat, low carb diet, higher digestion owing to the natural enzymes within the diet, Regularity within the movement since the diet is high in fiber, Lessens the chance of getting heart diseases and different diseases coupled to trans-fat and saturated fats within the food we tend to eat, Less water retention as a result of the diet is low in metal which implies it aids in maintaining a perfect weight, Protects against cancer since it's effective in cancer-fighting phytochemicals.

**Paleo Raw Food for Detoxing**

There is another important profit that may be gained with a Paleo Raw Food Diet - it rids the body of accumulated toxins. Toxins are harmful wastes or free radicals that are residues ensuing from breaking down food. they'll accumulate within the body through the years and harm cells which can even result in cancer. The body is unable to utterly disembarrass itself of those harmful toxins and through the time they accumulate to a degree that they hamper cell functions and have an effect on energy production and ultimately result in the event of diseases like cancer. feeding fiber-rich raw food diet helps the body get eliminate these toxins. Raw food diet contains antioxidants that neutralize the cell-damaging free radicals. It cleanses our organic process systems and fortifies the system.

# CHAPTER 9

## Formulating a recent Paleo Diet set up

Now that you just have a lot of or less a clearer understanding of the Paleo Diet, you've got to feel extremely driven to be able to adapt it to your lifestyle. And like every different nutritionary program, you've got to own an idea to place it into action. You can't simply dive in and play it by ear because it can solely result in failure and dismay. designing your switch to the Paleo lifestyle can guarantee your success as well as enable you to watch your progress. there's no "one size fits all" Paleo diet set up. each set up is unambiguously tailored to suit the wants and requirements of people. begin with a 28-day plan to eat solely Paleo food.

Below are some tips you'll be able to follow in formulating your planned transition to the Paleo modus vivendi.

Step one – take your beginning date. structure your mind once you wish the shift to begin and be firm regarding it. Don't take too long as you will get sidetracked by different things which will cause you to lose interest in it. Remember, it's your health and longevity at stake here.

Step two – Encourage members of the family to hitch in ever-changing over to the Paleo diet so you, therefore, won't be all by your lonesome self. Besides, with different members of the family within the same diet, you'd be able to inspire and facilitate one another out. it might be a fun and fulfilling journey the results of that are a few things everybody can care for for the remainder of their lives.

Step three – build a record of everything before you start on the program. Take measurements of yourself specifically your height and weight. See your doctor and have blood chemistry done on you to incorporate your blood sugars, CRP, pressure level, TG, HDL, LDL particle size, etc. All these can assist you to apprehend the sort of progress you're creating with the diet. And oh, don't forget to require an image of yourself with as very little garments on as doable. This may come in handy once examining you then and currently. write any health problems you will have before you begin on the diet. embody bloating, diarrhea, constipation, abdominal pain, acid reflux, gas, etc. this could complete the image of what you're before ever-changing over to the Paleo lifestyle.

Step four – free your room of all non-Paleo foodstuffs. Throw them away or to do better still, provide them intent on your neighbors. no matter you opt to try and do with them, make certain they're out of your sight and in a place wherever you can't be tempted to reach out for them.

Step five – go on a spree. Get your Paleo food list out and begin stocking upon them. Visit your friendly neighborhood foodstuff or grocery and if you can't notice some Paleo foodstuff there visit the farmers market. compose what you can't get from your nearest neighborhood food retailers and get them organized from on-line sources. The vital issue is to own everything Paleo in your room so you won't be tempted to use substitutes.

Step six – begin grouping Paleo Recipes and build a weekly design to last consecutive 28-day challenge. This way, you won't be at a loss on what to cook next.

Step seven – Don't take anybody's weight measurements until after the twenty-eight days. however fastidiously compose any physical or emotional changes you will feel within the course of the challenge. this manner you won't get frustrated if the changes are slow in returning. Don't worry, the changes can happen.

Step eight – in spite of what happens or no matter it's you are feeling stick with your set up till the last day of the 28-day challenge. At the top of the 28-day challenge, fastidiously measure the progress you've created if any. it's the time to seek out if the Paleo diet created you healthier, feel higher, change state, or if it worsened your condition instead.

**Evaluate by:**


Taking another image of yourself sporting constant garments once you took the primary picture. you'll be able to currently visually compare if there are variations between then and now. Take your body measurements over again and compare your weight and your region then and currently. Get another blood chemistry work done and raise your doctor's facilitate to interpret and compare the results then and currently. There will solely be one reason why the challenge won't bring the expected results. It should be as a result of you're not serious enough to strictly pursue the challenge to its completion and somewhere on the road, you've indulged in some exceptions or bust the diet from time to time.

If you don't notice any enhancements for currently, maybe your body wants longer to adapt to the new diet, therefore, stick with the diet a touch longer till there are manifest results. If you've achieved nice progress, then it's up to you to determine whether or not you ought to stick with the Paleo diet permanently.

Below may be a sample weekly Paleo design. You shouldn't have any problem with fashioning a weekly Paleo design. begin by grouping as many Paleo recipes as you'll be able to and selected people whom you fancy most. Incorporate them into a weekly design ensuring there's selection, therefore, you won't get bored consuming identical stuff over and over again. There are a lot of free online sources for Paleo diet recipes.

# CHAPTER 10

## Modern Paleo Principles

The modern Paleo diet is constructed upon the assumption that man's health and well being is maintained by intense a diet consisting of slightly processed food that was obtainable before the arrival of agriculture.

There are but no set of mounted rules very similar to commandments written on stone. everyone seems to be too liberal to eat the maximum amount as he desires as long as what he consumes belong to the Paleo food list as delineate within the previous chapters. There aren't any zones to follow, neither are there calories to count.

To a lot of avid Paleo advocates, the diet is straightforward enough to follow except for the primary time converts, the absence of set rules is confusing and should even tempt them to form excuses certainly exemptions currently then and break the diet to splurge on certain indulgences. For the inexperienced, we've listed below some pointers or recommendations on what to try to and what to not do. they're by no means that a group of rules to follow however a set of recommendations to guide you through your 1st Paleo journey.

Wheat, rice, corn, and all alternative grains don't have any place within the Paleo diet. they're no better than a sweetener.

Junk foods and restaurant food ready with edible fat and artificial food supplements also are out. you must eat real food instead.

Refined sugar, syrup, corn syrup, and artificial sweeteners are out.

Virgin coconut oil, nut oil, and vegetable oil along with side animal fats like butter, tallow, ghee, and lard are in. Refined oils like oil, edible fat, corn oil, and soy oil are out. change fats are out still.

Beans, legumes, peanuts, tubers, farm merchandise, don't have any place within the Paleo diet too.

Paleo is over a diet. it's a way of life which implies other than food, movement within the style of exercises and rest by the manner of sleeping are even as necessary. Together, food, sleep, and movement represent the 3 foundations of the fashionable Paleo lifestyle. Short, high-intensity daily exercises can have the best for the desired movement.

You should additionally make certain you get enough sleep a day. provide your body enough time to recover when every physical exertion. never abuse your body the least bit.

Avoid contact chemically the maximum amount as potential. Don't drink H2O. it's extremely chlorinated or fluoridated. Drink drinking water instead. With similar logic, avoid swimming in chlorinated pools.

Use solely deodorants that are freed from aluminum, halide-free dentifrice, and a lot of natural organic soap.

Do some intermittent abstinence 2 or 3 times per week. you'll skip breakfast and morning occasional. you may skip lunch too if you prefer. By fasting, you're starving the body cells to induce them to allocate the nutrients from cells that don't seem to be functioning optimally to be used to fuel alternative cell functions. you must not try this a day tho' because the body can learn to adapt to that negating the aim of abstinence.

You can save a great deal if you be a part of Community-supported agriculture programs. There should be one in your neighborhood or anyplace close to you. they're the most affordable supply of contemporary Paleo foodstuff. contemplate shopping for food in bulk like buying half a cow, or a bovid, or maybe a lamb rather than shopping for by the pound. you may save a great deal more this way. Besides, you may get all the prime cuts too. you may want a deep-freeze tho' for this and begin learning the way to cook shanks, shoulders, tails, trotters, and hocks. you may have been avoiding them within the past in favor of the prime cuts however you may be stunned at however delicious they taste. On prime of that, they sell cheaper that's why they're referred to as thrift cuts. you may save a large amount of cash together with them in your hotel plan.

Make it some extent to go to the farmer's market close to the top of the day and not an hour earlier. The farmers would need to urge to eliminate their merchandise before the day ends and are seeking to sell their turn out at a cut-price to anyone still hanging around the place instead of leaving them to waste.

Get organized. make certain you have got a Paleo searching list a weekly Paleo hotel plan. Check if all the Paleo ingredients for your weekly hotel plan are available. Being organizes from searching to change of state gets things done quicker and easier. you may additionally avoid shopping for too several things on impulse.

Make a minimum of a single day during a week your "Fish Day." On today eat solely no cooked fish like tuna fish salad with kippers for snacks with a great deal of raw inexperienced ivy-covered vegetables build use a great deal a part of your change of state. as an example, if you grill breast chicken these days, don't throw away the leftover. Store them within the white goods and use them for salad or fricassee every day or 2 later.

Don't be afraid to experiment change of state your meal from your Paleo instruction. try and produce one thing which will cause you to feel nice. There aren't any quick rules concerning making ready a Paleo meal as long as you keep on with the utilization of the Paleo food list. try and discover your vary of Paleo foods that cause you to feel nice and stick to it. Once again, don't be discouraged if you don't expertise immediate results. There are folks whose bodies want longer to regulate to a replacement diet. And don't be afraid if initially, you're feeling foggy or energetic. this can be a standard reaction once the body changes over to victimization fat for energy instead of from carbohydrates.

**CHAPTER 11**

**Paleo Diet for Athletes**

It is not solely those that have issues with their weight, or those searching for a cure for a few upset or unwellness who find the Paleo Diet healthfully useful. Even the able athletes within the peak of their form have found the Paleo to be the proper diet for them significantly the endurance athletes who usually pay several hours every day in intense coaching.

For years currently, biological process specialists are attempting to seem for that excellent food combination which will facilitate boost the athletes' endurance throughout coaching and guarantee wonderful performance during competitions. The biological process demand of the normal person who lives an inactive lifestyle is most a lot of differently from an athlete who is usually subjected to intense exertions virtually daily.

The Paleo diet seems to be a God-given gift to those champion athletes as most of them would attest to that. With the fashionable urban diet containing stuff that proves to be prohibitory to competitory athletes, nutritionists are scrambling to place along with a diet that's tailor-fitted to their specific biological process wants. As a result of that athletes bear intense workouts daily, Eat properly before, during, and when each physical exertion still as in between workouts is of overriding importance to confirm they need enough energy to realize peak performance and at a similar time facilitate their bodies recover quickly from the toilsome Exercise. the most focus of a perfect athlete's diet is to supply him with enough fuel to sustain him through several hours of intense energy output and to provide him nourishment when every session to assist the body recover quickly.

The ideal diet for endurance athletes should, therefore, be ready to do one issue - to keep up adequate glycemic masses within the blood the least bit times throughout the physical exertion. this could mean increasing saccharide consumption a lot of usually and in larger quantities than the traditional demand of the standard individual. Endurance athletes got to have a moderate intake of carbohydrates 2 hours before every intense physical exertion. this can provide the body enough time to bring the blood glucose to the suitable levels suited to rigorous exertions that need intense energy output. If the workouts are aiming to be tedious, the athlete might need to increase his saccharide intake often throughout the length of the exercise. For workouts that last no over an hour, water often would satisfy.

He should additionally eat foods wealthy in carbohydrates and with a modest quantity of supermolecule at intervals the primary 30 minutes when every physical exertion. this can be essential for quick and effective recovery. If necessary, he will continue intense high saccharide foods for many hours for an extended recovery. After this, he should return to his regular Paleo diet program. The nutrient demand of an athlete might vary from time to time looking at his coaching schedule. The saccharide and fat intake as shown described above schedule is meant to travel on well with the opposing swings in the athlete's energy utilization because the coaching progresses from totally different stages. it's vital to notice down these energy swings and program the saccharide and supermolecule intake consequently.

The Paleo Diet is, of course, Ergogenic maybe the foremost important feature of the Paleo Diet that specifically edges athletes is it being ergogenic. It means that it's packed with nutrients that enhance the performance of athletes. it's significantly high in animal supermolecule that is that the best supply of branched-chain amino acids like essential amino acid, valine, an essential amino acid that is liable for muscle growth and repair. the fashionable urban diet is often acidic and therefore the body's natural reaction to neutralize acidity by breaking down muscle tissues. Athletes on a Western diet unremarkably would realize it hard to keep up and enhance their muscle stores when a tough day's physical exertion. On the opposite hand, athletes on the Paleo Diet don't suffer supermolecule breakdown in their muscle mass. The Paleo diet produces a net alkalic result within the body that is that the actual opposite of what the up to date Western diet produces. This eliminates the requirement for the supermolecule-breaking reaction of the body to acidic diets, therefore, no protein muscle breakdown happens. The Paleo Diet for athletes needs to be changed to'. It should be tailored specifically to an athlete's coaching program and nutrient needs. It should be changed in such a manner that permits a tiny low window of chance for the consumption of starches and straightforward sugars by the athletes from non-Paleo sources throughout, before, and after the particular exercise. It should allow high carbo intake by athletes as required and once it suits them best whereas coaching each to stay them in their peak forms throughout the physical exertion session and to provide them the much-needed nutrients for his or her bodies to recover quickly in time for subsequent arduous exercise.

Outside of the coaching schedule, it's strictly Paleo all the manner – low carb, high supermolecule diet. which means intense loads of lean meat, seafood, poultry, vegetables, and contemporary fruits as much because the athletes like. To summarize, the Paleo Diet has the subsequent useful benefits for athletes as Compared to alternative diets accessible nowadays for endurance athletes: The Paleo diet for athletes has a lot of the open-chain amino acids which boosts muscle growth and anabolic perform. The Branched-chain amino acids conjointly stop or minimize the suppression of the system that ordinarily follows intensive workouts by endurance athletes.

The diet strikes a balance between the inflammation inflicting omega6 fatty acids and useful omega3 fatty acids. It reduces if not eliminates post-workout tissue inflammations that usually affect athletes once a strenuous physical exercise. The Paleo diet produces an alkalic result that lowers the body's acidity so reducing the debilitating effect of pathology on the bones and muscles whereas at a similar time causing supermolecule synthesis within the muscle tissues for a lot of muscle growth. The Paleo Diet includes nutrient-rich vegetables and food. they're filled with essential vitamins and trace minerals required by endurance athletes to take care of optimum health and for effective future recovery from hard exercises.

Training for such endurance sports as running, weight lifting, cycling, swimming, triathlon, rowing, and race marathons is onerous to the body. The endurance athlete is consistently in some variety of a recovery stage following each strenuous physical exercise. this can be wherever the Paleo diet is important to an athlete because it re-nourishes the body with the much-needed carbohydrates and proteins it lost within the coaching whereas at a similar time providing the body with trace nutrients and vitamins required to repair the body back to type. Together, the Paleo diet and a very quiet sleep become the essential elements of the endurance athlete's educational program.

The athlete must recover quickly and effectively once every serious physical exercise for him to be prepared and ready for succeeding. This has invariably been the largest challenge an endurance athlete faces in preparation for a contest. Let the reality be told, it'll be not possible for an athlete to form a full and quick recovery with a strictly all Paleo diet. What he consumes ought to be ready to make full the stored nutrients and polyose he lost on every coaching session and an occasional carb high supermolecule diet just like the Paleo diet won't fulfill as it is. that's why the Paleo diet must be changed to incorporate the employment of non-Paleo high sugar sources throughout, prior, and post-training. it's the sole way to guarantee speedy recovery in time for succeeding serious calculate. In short, a changed Paleo diet for jocks must be developed to accommodate all the nutrient needs of an endurance athlete.

**Formulating the Paleo Diet for Athletes**

As has been realized earlier, the Paleo diet must be slightly changed to suit the necessities of endurance athletes on coaching. Specifically, they have to enhance their sugar intake at totally different stages of every serious physical exercise. Before the physical exercise, sugar intake is required to boost the sugar load within the blood to a suitable level for the expected intense energy output. High sugar intake throughout the physical exercise is additionally necessary to take care of peak performance. And to be ready to recover quickly from the hard physical exercise, sugar intake is once more required within the initial few hours in real-time following the physical exercise to assist the body recover quickly and be prepared for succeeding. Again, the modifications ought to be slight and temporary long enough to last the length of the coaching period. There are not any quick and firm rules on however one ought to move it. It shouldn't, however, veer away too far away from the fundamental Paleo ideas.

Below are some basic Paleo Principles you'll be able to use in customizing your Paleo diet for athletes:

Leave out all processed foods from your food list and eat solely natural organic foods. Processed foods have artificial ingredients that will impact your body chemistry and have an effect on your performance furthermore as your health.

Make fruits and vegetables, haywire and seeds, as your main supply of carbohydrates. Limit your consumption of sugary energy drink supplements to coaching sessions. Take them solely as required however avoid them for the remainder of the day.

20 to 25th of your calorie demand should be from animal supermolecule significantly from grass-fed farm animal and poultry, game meats and from non-farmed fish and food.

Increase your consumption of fish and walnuts and alternative sources of omega-three fatty acids to balance the presence of inflammation inflicting omega-six from other food sources.

Don't eat food cooked with trans fat like canola, corn, and soy oil. If you wish to fry food use vegetable oil or virgin oil instead. It is much better to don't fry, grill or broil instead. Processed snack foods are high in trans fats, therefore, avoid them too. you furthermore might need to limit your consumption of saturated fats.

**Leave out all dairy farm merchandise from your diet.**

**Drink an abundance of water. keep it your main fluid intake.**

Other a lot of specific modifications on the Paleo diet for athletes can depend upon the character of the game, the volume, and intensity of the coaching furthermore as on the physical build of the athlete. Generally, the larger the athlete is, or the tougher or longer the coaching, a lot of carbohydrates are required - before, during, and after the physical exercise.

Power athletes like sprinters, weight lifters, football players, and swimmers, as an example, need to consume one gram of supermolecule per pound of weight during a day as a general rule. Others have benefited enormously from what Doctor Mauro Di- Pasquale calls a 'cyclical low sugar diet' wherever they get to consume higher carbohydrate intake once or double per week solely to condition the body to burn fat for fuel too. Dr. Di-Pasquale could be a recognized authority on dietary regimens for athletes.

# CHAPTER 12

## PALEO RECIPES

PALEO BREAKFAST RECIPES

## FROM THE GARDEN BASIL CHICKEN SALAD

Ingredients:

2 enormous destroyed, and pre-cooked skinless chicken bosoms

2 little pitted avocados

1/3 cup de-stemmed basil leaves

2 ½ tbsp. olive oil

¼ tsp. dark pepper

¼ tsp. ocean salt

Directions:

Start by situating the destroyed chicken in your blending bowl. Next, include the olive oil, the avocado, the basil, the salt, and the pepper to a food processor. Heartbeat the fixings until they're smooth. Add this blend over the destroyed chicken and hurl the chicken well to coat it completely. Season the chicken to taste, and enable it to rest in the refrigerator before serving.

## CHINESE-BASED CABBAGE CHICKEN SALAD

Ingredients:

1 ¾ cup hacked and cooked chicken

4 cups chopped savoy cabbage 1/3 cup

1/3 cup julienned scallions

1 cup julienned carrot

1/3 cup packed cilantro

1/3 cup julienned radishes 1/3 cup hacked mint

Dressing Ingredients:

2 tbsp. sesame oil

2 ¼ tbsp. coconut vinegar

2 ½ tbsp. coconut aminos

1 diced chipotle pepper

juice from ½ lime

1 tsp. nectar

3 minced garlic cloves

1 tsp. diced ginger

Directions:

Start by combining the hacked and julienned carrots, cabbage, scallions, what's more, radishes. Include the mint, the cilantro, and the slashed chicken, and hurl the plate of mixed greens in an enormous blending bowl. Next, position the serving of mixed greens to the side. To make the vinaigrette, start by expelling the chipotle pepper seeds. Spread the pepper with water and enable it to sit for thirty minutes.

Following thirty minutes, add the pepper to the sustenance processor and heartbeat it for one minute before adding different fixings to the processor. Taste the vinaigrette, what's more, change the flavors if you please. Pour the dressing over the made serving of mixed greens, and prepare the plate of mixed greens to coat.

## MEXICAN-INSPIRED CHICKEN TACO SALAD

Ingredients:

2 tbsp. taco flavoring (made beneath)

½ pound destroyed chicken

1/3 cup water

1 tbsp. olive oil

1 head destroyed lettuce

1 diced tomato

1 diced red onion

1 little, hollowed avocado

½ diced green pepper

Directions:

**Start by combining the taco flavoring, as followings.**

Unite 1 tsp. garlic powder, 4 tbsp. bean stew powder, 2 tsp. paprika 1 tsp. onion powder 1 tsp. oregano, ¼ tsp. red pepper pieces, 3 tsp. salt Blend the fixings before taking out the 2 tbsp. of the taco flavoring you require for this formula. (Note that you can keep the flavoring for a later formula if you so pick.) Next, heat the olive oil in the skillet. Add the chicken to the olive oil to give it an increase in flavor. Pour the water over top, alongside the taco flavoring. Enable the chicken blend to stew until the water vanishes. Next, cut up the various fixings. Make the serving of mixed greens by amassing together the vegetables, the chicken, and so forth. Hurl the fixings well, and appreciate it!

**AVOCADO-BASED PALEO CHICKEN SALAD**

Ingredients:

3 skinless and boneless chicken bosoms, pre-cooked and destroyed

1/3 diced onion

1 diced avocado

2 tbsp. lime juice

3 tbsp. cilantro

salt and pepper to taste

Directions:

Bring all the above fixings together and blend well, making a point to crush the avocado as you go. Enjoy this exceptionally straightforward formula.

Muffins made up of Almond Flour

Ingredients:

1 cup blanched almond flour (4 oz)

two eggs

one tbsp century plant nectar or honey

¼ tsp hydrogen carbonate

½ tsp apple vinegar

Instructions:

Combine almond flour and hydrogen carbonate in an exceedingly medium-size bowl. combine the eggs, agave, and vinegar in an exceedingly larger bowl Cut within the dry ingredients into the egg mixture, mix well till the material is consistent. Scoop batter into a paper-lined quick bread pan ¼ cup at a time. Heat kitchen appliance to 350° and bake muffins for quarter-hour or till the perimeters are slightly tanned Cool the muffins whereas still within the pan for a minimum of half an hour. Add butter and raspberry jam

Makes four muffins. You can use identical ingredients and therefore the same directions to form a fast bread loaf. simply double the ingredients and bake it longer – forty to forty-five minutes rather than quarter-hour. Use a little loaf pan.

**PALEO NUTTY BARS FOR BREAKFAST**

Ingredients:

1 Cup almond flour ( blanched)

¼ tsp kosher salt

two tbsp honey

¼ C copra oil, one tbsp water

½ Cup sliced coconut ( unsweetened)

¼ Craisins

½ Cup pumpkin seeds

¼ Cup almonds (blanched slivered

one tsp seasoning

½ Cup flower seeds

Instructions:

Combine and blend salt and almond flour in a baking oven. Cut in water, honey, copra oil, and vanilla. Add cut coconut, almond slivers, raisins, pumpkin seeds, and flower seeds.

Place the dough firmly into a regular baking pan, and pat down the dough utilizing your hands wet with water. Bake for twenty minutes at 350°.

## PALEO PORRIDGE

Ingredients:

two mashed bananas

a pair of Cup coconut milk

1/4 cup flax meal

3/4 cup almond meal

one tsp cinnamon

1/8 tsp ground cloves

1/2 tsp ginger

1/8 tsp ground nutmeg

syrup or raw honey as the sweetener

1/8 tsp coarse ocean salt

You may add unsweetened coconut flakes berries, nuts, or seeds, for topping.

Instructions:

Use a medium-size pan. place altogether the ingredients and simmer on low heat. Stir often till thick and produces bubbles. it'll be at the start skinny however will bite by bit thicken as you cook. it'll thicken therefore a lot of when cookery until up to serving time so it's best that you simply add a bit further coconut milk or water. high with berries or coconut flakes before serving.

## KALE SALAD

Ingredients:

1 few kale leaves, three ounces Andouille sausage, 1/2 cup sliced mushrooms, ½ cup diced onion, one/4 cup + 1 tablespoon further virgin oil, a pair of tbsp apple vinegar, one tsp + a lot of to style, 1/2 tsp cracked black pepper, a pair of eggs deep-fried.

Instructions:

Slice the kale leaves by removing the stalks and dense spines. Rinse, and pat dry thoroughly. Dice the kale leaves into bite-sized pieces, put away in a big blender. Cut the Andouille sausage and cook on medium fire one tablespoon of the oil and a medium-sized frypan. Cook sausage till a lot of the fat has been taken out and consequently the sausage is somewhat crisp. Add the mushrooms and onions and simmer for five more minutes. Lower the heat and add a quarter cup of oil in conjunction with pepper, salt, and apple vinegar. Stir well for some seconds till everything is heated through. Pour the still-hot Andouille sausage dressing over the kale and put away. Fry 2 eggs. Throw the dish with the dressing and divide among 2 plates. Serve the dish with the egg on top of it.

PALEO LUNCH RECIPES

## Beef Barbacoa

Ingredients:

Six pounds small beef roast cuts

eight garlic cloves

six slices chipotle peppers

six peppers

one tbsp dried oregano

three tbsp coconut oil

two tbsp ground cumin

one tablespoon black pepper powder

five bay leaves

one tbsp Kosher salt

half cup of apple vinegar

six tablespoons of lime juice

1 teaspoon of cloves

ground 1 1/2 cups beef stock

two pieces of juniper berries.


Instructions:


Heat two tbsp of oil on a medium heat using a large pan. Pan Fry each side of the meat for about two to three minutes making sure they are cooked or properly browned. Place the lightly tanned meat in a Crockpot.

Put the vinegar, adobo sauce, chipotle peppers, garlic, oregano, lime juice, cumin, salt, black pepper, and cloves in a food blender and mix until it is smooth. Pour blended sauce over meat and then add the beef stock and then garnish the top of the meat.

Cover the crockpot and use a low flame to cook for six hours until the meat is very tender. Transfer the liquid into a wide bottom pan and let simmer on high heat until the quantity is reduced by only one half of the original quantity.


**Paleo Chicken Fajitas**


Ingredients:

3 pounds sliced chicken breast piece

three sliced onions

three bell peppers

five garlic cloves(finely chopped)

lemon juice (four lemons)

three tablespoons each of oregano

cumin, coriander and chili powder

four tablespoons of coconut oil

lettuce leaves and butter for serving the fajitas

You have the choice for your fajita toppings. It can anything from chopped tomatoes, sliced avocados, pickles, guacamole, sauerkraut, and mayonnaise.

Instructions:

Blend the onions, chicken, bell peppers, garlic and spices in a blender. Mix them well inside the blender and put the mixture in the white sauce to infuse it for four hours, take a big enough fry pan and heat it under low flame and add the oil. Put the chicken that is marinated into the frypan and cook the bell peppers and onion are crisp and also the chicken is completely prepared. Now, transfer the chicken and veggies mixture into a large enough bowl and now to make a fajita with placing the lettuce leaves and top it any of the veggies garnish.

**Garlic mussels with White Wine**

Ingredients:

four lbs new mussels

two chopped onions

five finely hacked cloves garlic

two cups white wine or chicken stock

six tbsp spread or ghee

1/3 cup of your preferred herbs.

Directions:

Wash the mussels altogether and clean its hair. Discard the majority of the opened mussels cooking. Utilize a stockpot for cooking. Spot the white wine, garlic and onions and heat to the point of boiling. Stew for around 5 minutes before including the cleaned mussels. Spread and raise the temperature to medium-high. Give it a chance to bubble until every one of the mussels is open. Include the herbs and spread (or ghee) before expelling the pot from the flame. Serve in dishes with margarine sauce, white wine, and garlic.

**Pork slashes with apples and onions**

Ingredients:

Four pork slashes bone-in and with trimmings

two enormous onion(sliced)

three tbsp crude margarine

four apples(cut with the center removed)

Pepper and Salt.

Guidelines:

Rub the pork slashes with salt and pepper. Spot a huge dish on a stove over medium-high warmth and soften two tablespoons of your favored cooking fat. Sear each side of the pork hacks for five minutes or until caramelized and appropriately cooked. Put in a safe spot for some time. Set the warmth among medium and low at that point include the rest of the 1 tablespoon of fat. Include apple cuts and cut onions. Cook for at any rate four minutes or until the apple cuts are somewhat delicate and the onions have all the earmarks of being as of now caramelized. Top the pork slashes with cooked apple cuts and onions and serve.

**Gluten-Free Chicken Strips**

Ingredients:

1/2 lbs. boneless chicken chest parts

1 tbsp grapeseed oil

⅓ C coconut oil

½ cup coconut flour

¾ cup destroyed coconut

½ tsp salt

12 pounds crisp black pepper

1 egg

Guidelines:

Set the broiler temperature at 4000 F. While preheating the broiler, set up the flour blend. Consolidate flour with pepper and salt in a blending bowl (medium size). Beat the egg together with 1 tbsp of grapeseed oil in a different bowl. Spot the precut coconut in another bowl. Plunge the chicken pieces first in the flour blend ensuring each piece is covered equitably. Plunge the chicken pieces into the egg blend than on the destroyed coconut. Organize the covered chicken pieces in a low sided heating container and shower with coconut oil or softened spread. Heat for fifteen to twenty minutes turning the chicken over once.

## Basic Shrimp Scampi

Ingredients:

1 lb of shrimp or prawns

3 tbsp field margarine or ghee

3 cloves of garlic (finely slashed)

1/2 lemon squeezed

Salt and Pepper

Guidelines:

Warm your griddle first before including the margarine. When the skillet is hot enough diminish the warmth to medium-low and include the margarine. Include the garlic once the margarine is dissolved. Include the recently washed and dried shrimps. Sauté the shrimps for 10 minutes or until they are never again translucent. Expel from the flame and include the lemon juice. Raced with some salt and pepper before serving hot.

## Broiled Chicken with Citrus and Garlic

Ingredients:

1 entire chicken

1 cup onion iodized salt

1 orange

Some water to cover the feathered creature in a stockpot

Roasting the Chicken

1 stick field spread

cut into 1 inch thick cuts

1 lemon

1 huge orange

3 sprigs rosemary finely chopped

6 cloves garlic finely chopped

Barely any drops of Extra Virgin Olive Oil

Guidelines:

**Brining the Chicken**

Evacuate the giblets and put the chicken in a huge stockpot and spread with water. Heat some water in a different container including one cup of salt until all the salt is broken up. Include the bubbled salted water together with the squeezed orange (incorporate the skin) to the huge stockpot with chicken and permit to marinate for at least 3 hours or maybe even close to 5 hours inside the fridge.

**Broiling the Chicken**

Preheat the stove to 425. Gently wash the marinated chicken and pat dry. With your fingers, make a 'spread pocket' by isolating the chicken skin from the bosoms. Spot the spread cuts to the 'margarine pockets' under the skin together with half of the hacked garlic.

Addition the oranges, lemons, the rest of the garlic and rosemary inside the chicken cavity. Leave some rosemary for embellishing. Brush the skin of the chicken with a little olive oil at that point sprinkle with the leftover rosemary.

Cook the chicken at 425 degrees for 90 minutes. In the wake of broiling the chicken haul it out of the stove and brush the outside skin with liquefied margarine in the heating container. Cut and serve.

## Paleo Chicken Salad Wraps

Ingredients:

1/2 cup cleaved cooked or bubbled chicken

3 tbsp cleaved Fuji apples

2 tbsp cleaved red grapes

2 tsp nectar

2 tbsp almond margarine

Guidelines:

Make a simple Paleo chicken serving of mixed greens by combining all fixings. Envelop the chicken plate of mixed greens by a Romaine leaf and serve.

## Paleo Nutty Meatloaf Recipe

Ingredients:

1 lb ground meat

5 cloves garlic, minced

1 little green pepper finely hacked

1 tsp basil finely grounded

1 tsp rosemary finely grounded

1 tsp thyme finely grounded

A ½ cup of blended ground almonds, pecans, and walnuts

2 eggs

Black pepper, ground

Directions:

Put every one of the fixings in a major blending bowl. Make sure the fixings are uniformly joined in the blend. Spot the blend in the fridge for 30 minutes to 60 minutes. Oil a portion container utilizing olive oil and move the blend into it. Heat for one hour and 15 minutes. Cut and serve.

**Paleo Steak with Mushroom and Onion Gravy**

Ingredients:

3 pieces 6-ounce Sirloin steak

1 cup of coconut milk

2 tbsp coconut flour

1 medium onion cut

2 to 3 garlic cloves squashed

1/8 tsp cayenne pepper

1/4 tsp ocean salt

1/2 cup cut mushrooms

1/2 tsp dark pepper

1 tbsp coconut oil

Directions:

Setting up the Steaks:

Sear, flame broil, or sauté the steak to your favored doneness.

**Setting up the Gravy:**

Coat a skillet with cooking oil and warmth at a high setting. Blend in onions, mushrooms, and garlic. Whenever delicate, expel from the skillet and set it aside a short time. Include the coconut flour into the skillet and blend in the coconut milk.

Keep blending at high warmth until the blend is smooth. Diminish the warmth when the blend is smooth and include the flavoring. Add the vegetable to the now practically thick sauce. Stew for another 5 to 10 minutes. Coat the cooked steaks with the thick sauce liberally and serve.

**Paleo Pot Roast**

Ingredients:

3 pounds rear end cook, with the fat cut

2 tbsp coconut oil

1 onion, enormous, chopped

2 celery ribs, cleaved

1/2 tbsp dried thyme

3 cloves garlic, minced

2 C hamburger soup (without additive)

1/2 tsp dried parsley

1 to 2 straight leaves

20 entire peppercorns

1/2 tbsp ocean salt

6 to 7 florets of cauliflower

2 carrots, cut

1/3 C coconut flour

1/2 tsp ocean salt

Directions:

Warmth coconut oil on a Dutch broiler or any thick-walled cooking pot. Include the back end broil and burn all sides. Expel the dish from the Dutch broiler and put it in a platter. Put the celery, parsley, onion, thyme, and garlic into the Dutch broiler and sauté for 5 minutes; Put the burned posterior meal back to the Dutch stove.

Include the stock, sound leaf, ocean salt and peppercorns. Spread and spot inside the broiler preheated to 3250 F. Cook the dish for 4 hours treating it each half-hour. Evacuate broil after it is done and strain the stock into a bowl. Discard the vegetables keeping just the stock. Shred the meat with the utilization of two forks and put the destroyed meat again into the Dutch broiler.

Submerge the destroyed hamburger with the recently stressed fluid from the pot. Toss in the cauliflower, carrots and the rest of the ocean salt. Put inside the stove again and stew for an additional 45 minutes. Channel the stock from the Dutch broiler and measure. Include more hamburger juices on the off chance that important to make 3 cups of stock, at that point empty every one of the 3 cups into the pot. Mix in the flour and stew until it transforms into a thick sauce. Spread the meat and vegetables with the sauce.

**Beef Roll**

Ingredients:

1 ½ pound ground beef

1 egg

½ red or white onion (stripped and diced)

Dark pepper and salt to taste

½ tbsp olive oil

1/8 cup finely diced parsley

Directions:

Beat egg well in a little bowl and put in a safe spot. In a different bowl blend the ground hamburger with diced onion, pepper and salt. Include the egg into the meat blend and blend well. Fold parts of the meat blend into medium frankfurter sizes.

Line sauce skillet with olive oil and warmth at medium-high. Include each hamburger roll and flame broil until completely dark-colored everywhere. Expel the meat moves from the container and spot on a plate secured with a paper towel. Give it a chance to remain until the abundance fat channel. Organize the hamburger moves over your preferred vegetable. Brimming with new parsley drops and serve.

## Shrimp, Cantaloupe and Mint Salad

Fixings:

3 C crisp Arugula

1 C ready mango solid shapes

crisp 1/2 lbs.

medium shrimps pre-cooked

3 tbsp Crisp lemon juice

1 Cup melon 3D squares

new 1 tsp nutmeg

1 tsp cinnamon

Directions:

Blend shrimp, melon, mango, nutmeg, cinnamon, and lemon juice. Top the plate of mixed greens blend with your decision of balsamic dressing. To set up the Balsamic Dressing: Combine olive oil, nectar and balsamic vinegar in a bowl. Serves 4

## Paleo Grilled Salmon with Asparagus

Fixings:

1 lb salmon

1/2 lb cherry tomatoes

1/2 lb asparagus

1 tsp ocean salt

1 tbsp olive oil

1 tsp dark pepper

Fixings:

Line a skillet with olive oil and sauté until delicate the cut asparagus. Add pepper and salt to taste. Put in a safe spot while you set up the salmon. Clean crisp salmon and season as indicated by your taste. Sear salmon ensuring it is completely cooked start to finish. When cooked expel salmon from skillet and put in a safe spot. Spot the sautéed asparagus on a serving plate and spot the cooked salmon over it. Trimming with ½ lb cherry tomatoes and serve.

**Paleo Chicken Stir Fry**

Fixings:

1 lb boneless chicken cutlets

1/2 lb broccoli florets

5 cloves garlic finely cleaved

1/4 lb red ringer peppers (cut)

2 tbsp coconut oil

1/4 lb crisp carrots

1/4 lb finely cleaved chives

ocean salt and dark pepper to taste

Guidelines:

Put a little coconut oil to a fricasseeing and sauté chicken cutlets until seared and cooked all together. Put the cooked chicken cutlets aside. Warmth coconut oil in another griddle. Include the broccoli, carrots, red pepper, garlic and chives. Stew until the vegetables are delicate. Include the chicken cutlets and season with pepper and salt to taste. Spot in a serving plate and serve.

**Heated Chicken with Pomegranate Glaze**

Ingredients:

1 entire chicken (around 4 to 5 lbs)

1 enormous lemon (punctured with a fork)

1 tbsp Dijon mustard

2 sprigs rosemary, new

Seeds from 1 pomegranate

1 tbsp finely slashed garlic

2 sprigs crisp thyme

2 cups pomegranate juice, unsweetened 2 tbsp in addition to 1 tsp arrowroot

1 tsp nectar

1/2 ocean salt 1/2 tsp newly ground dark pepper

Directions:

Spot punctured lemon and rosemary inside the chicken hole. Tie the chicken legs together to keep it firm and set in a cooking skillet. Combine pomegranate juice, mustard, thyme, arrowroot, and garlic for treating. Pour the blend everywhere throughout the chicken and sprinkle with salt and pepper. Spot inside a stove preheated to 375 degrees. Prepare for 25 minutes. Take it out and season the chicken.

Prepare for an additional 25 minutes and afterward treat once more. Include the pomegranate seeds and diminish stove temperature to 350 degrees Fahrenheit. Bake for one more hour while seasoning each half-hour this time. At the point when done deplete the fluid and put in a safe spot. Spread the chicken with foil and let it represent 30 minutes. Serve the chicken with the coating.

**Paleo Roasted Chicken and Herbal Gravy**

Ingredients:

5 to 6 boneless chicken bosom (with skin)

1/2 tsp dried thyme

1-quart natural low sodium chicken juices

2 tbsp crisp rosemary (sprigs)

4 to 5 tbsp olive oil or coconut oil

8 squashed garlic cloves

2 to 3 tbsp coconut flour or almond flour.

ocean salt and pepper to taste

Directions:

Spread chicken bosoms with olive oil and season with pepper and salt. Mastermind in a preparing sheet that has been fixed with aluminum foil. Spot inside the broiler preheated to 350 degrees. Heat without spread until the chicken is cooked (around 30 minutes). Remove it from the broiler and cut the chicken bosoms on a level plane into 2-inch cuts.

**For the Gravy**

Warmth coconut oil in a sauce skillet over high warmth. Pour in the chicken stock, thyme, rosemary, salt, pepper, and garlic. Blend well and steadily lessen warmth to low. Keep on stewing until you have the ideal surface and consistency. Spot cook chicken bosom, blend well, and afterward expel from flame. Serve hot.

**Paleo Pumpkin and Chicken Curry**

Ingredients:

2 pieces sliced chicken breasts

2 tablespoon olive oil

5 cups pumpkin, diced

2 garlic cloves, finely chopped

1 bunch fresh coriander

chopped 1 onion, diced

2 tbsp ginger, ground

1 tbsp turmeric, ground

2 tbsp coriander, ground

2 tbsp cumin, ground

1 ½ cups vegetable stock Salt

Instructions:

**Sauté garlic and onion in a Frypan for two minutes over medium heat.**

Add chicken and simmer while stirring frequently for ten minutes until chicken turns white. Stir in the pumpkin, cumin, turmeric, ginger, and coriander and continue to stir for one minute. Pour the vegetable stock and simmer for 15minutes on low heat. Stir in the chopped coriander then put the cover on and simmer for another two minutes. Add salt to taste.

Egg and Capsicum Salad

Ingredients:

2 eggs, hard-boiled, diced

1tbsp coconut oil

2 diced bacon eyes

½ diced green capsicum

¼ C slashed parsley

1tbsp mayonnaise

1 C serving of mixed greens leaves, blended

Procedure:

Cook bacon in a coconut oil covered griddle over medium warmth. Broil the bacon until it begins to be fresh. Channel the abundance oil and move the bacon to a bowl. Include the bubbled eggs, parsley, capsicum, and mayonnaise. Hurl well. Orchestrate the plate of mixed greens on a serving plate and top with egg and capsicum blend to serve.

**Prepared Chicken with Pomegranate Glaze**

Ingredients:

1 entire chicken (around 4 to 5 lbs)

1 huge lemon (punctured with a fork)

1 tbsp Dijon mustard

2 sprigs rosemary, new

Seeds from 1 pomegranate

1 tbsp finely chopped garlic

2 sprigs new thyme

2 cups pomegranate juice unsweetened

2 tbsp in addition to 1 tsp arrowroot

1 tsp nectar

1/2 ocean salt

1/2 tsp newly ground dark pepper

Directions:

Spot punctured lemon and rosemary inside the chicken pit. Tie the chicken legs together to keep it firm and set in a simmering dish. Blend pomegranate juice, mustard, thyme, arrowroot, and garlic for seasoning. Pour the blend everywhere throughout the chicken and sprinkle with salt and pepper. Spot inside a stove preheated to 375 degrees. Heat for 25 minutes. Take it out and treat the chicken. Heat for an additional 25 minutes and afterward treat once more. Include the pomegranate seeds and diminish stove temperature to 350 degrees Fahrenheit. Heat for one more hour while treating each half-hour this time. At the point when done deplete the fluid and put in a safe spot. Spread the chicken with foil and let it represent 30 minutes. Serve the chicken with the coating.

**Paleo Roasted Chicken and Herbal Gravy**

Ingredients:

5 to 6 boneless chicken bosom (with skin)

1/2 tsp dried thyme

1-quart natural low sodium chicken stock

2 tbsp crisp rosemary (sprigs)

4 to 5 tbsp olive oil or coconut oil

8 squashed garlic cloves

2 to 3 tbsp coconut flour or almond flour.

Ocean salt and pepper to taste

Guidelines:

Spread chicken bosoms with olive oil and season with pepper and salt. Organize in a preparing sheet that has been fixed with aluminum foil. Spot inside the stove preheated to 350 degrees. Heat without spread until the chicken is cooked (around 30 minutes). Remove it from the stove and cut the chicken bosoms on a level plane into 2-inch cuts.

For the Gravy

Warmth coconut oil in a sauce container over high warmth. Pour in the chicken soup, thyme, rosemary, salt, pepper, and garlic. Blend well and progressively lessen warmth to low. Keep on stewing until you have the ideal surface and consistency. Spot broil chicken bosom, blend well, and after that expel from flame. Serve hot.

**Paleo Pumpkin and Chicken Curry**

Ingredients:

2 pieces cut chicken bosoms

2 tablespoon olive oil

5 cups pumpkin, diced

2 garlic cloves, finely cleaved

1 bundle new coriander, chopped

1 onion, diced

2 tbsp ginger, ground

1 tbsp turmeric, ground

2 tbsp coriander, ground

2 tbsp cumin, ground

1 ½ cups vegetable stock Salt

Guidelines:

Sauté garlic and onion in a Fry search for gold minutes over medium warmth. Include chicken and stew while blending regularly for ten minutes until chicken turns white. Blend in the pumpkin, cumin, turmeric, ginger, and coriander and keep on mixing for one moment. Pour the vegetable stock and stew for 15minutes on low warmth. Mix in the hacked coriander at that point put the spread on and stew for an additional two minutes. Add salt to taste.

**Paleo Crispy Orange Chicken**

Ingredients:

2 pounds chicken (deboned, skinless )

1/4 tsp pepper

1.5 tsp ocean salt

.5 Cup coconut feast/flour

1 tbsp coconut oil, additional virgin

1 egg

For the Glaze:

1 teaspoon garlic, minced

1 cup crisp squeezed orange

1.5 tsp ground orange skin

1.5 C hoisin sauce

1/4 cup nectar

Dash of cayenne pepper Sea Salt Pepper

Guidelines:

Cut the chicken into two-inch pieces and spot them in an enormous compartment or a blending bowl. Include the egg, coconut oil, pepper and ocean salt. Join well and set aside. Put the ½ cup coconut supper/flour blend in a different bowl and plunge the chicken on the flour blend ensuring each piece is covered liberally.

Get enough coconut oil to fill a big fry pan to about half an inch from its base. Put the frying pan on the stove and set the temperature on high warmth until it achieves 3750 F. Begin singing the chicken pieces by groups. Broil each cluster until the chicken cutlets are sautéed, fresh, and crunchy. This ought to be around 3-4 minutes for each cluster. Take out the chicken pieces from the skillet and channel them well over paper towels.

Wrap up the remainder of the chicken pieces and put them in a safe spot while you set up the coating. Expel all the oil from the skillet leaving just around 2 tbsp. of oil and lower the temperature to medium warmth.

Sauté the garlic for one moment however abstain from consuming it else it will give a harsh taste. Hurl in the various fixings and let the blend bubble. Blend the bubbling blend for three minutes before decreasing the warmth. Keep on stewing the blend until you produce the coating. Spread the chicken with the coating and enrich with chives and orange cuts before serving.

**Stovetop Spring Frittata**

Ingredients:

1 tablespoon olive oil

1 clove garlic minced

1 radish ground or finely cleaved

1/2 cup cleaved asparagus

3 eggs beaten

1 teaspoon crisp slashed mint

Ocean salt and crisp ground pepper to taste

Guidelines:

Warmth the oil in a little skillet over medium-low warmth. Include the garlic, radish, and asparagus and cook until relaxed. Season with salt and pepper. Include the eggs and cook for a moment until the edges are set. Lift the edges cautiously and let the fluid stream underneath the edges. Turn the warmth down to low and cover the container. Cook for 2-3 minutes until eggs are cooked through. Top with the crisp mint.

**Egg and Capsicum Salad**

Ingredients:

2 eggs, hard-boiled, diced

1tbsp coconut oil

2 diced bacon eyes

½ diced green capsicum

¼ C slashed parsley

1tbsp mayonnaise

A cup serving of mixed greens leaves, blended

Guidelines:

Cook bacon in a coconut oil covered griddle over medium warmth. Broil the bacon until it begins to be firm. Channel the abundance oil and move the bacon to a bowl. Include the bubbled eggs, parsley, capsicum, and mayonnaise. Hurl well. Orchestrate the serving of mixed greens on a serving plate and top with egg and capsicum blend to serve.

Paleo bread recipes

## Date and Walnut Bread

Ingredients:

½ C almond flour, whitened
2 tbsp coconut flour
¼ tsp heating soft drink
⅛ tsp Celtic ocean salt
3 enormous Medjool dates
1 tbsp apple juice vinegar
3 eggs
½ cup pecans, slashed

Guidelines:

With a sustenance processor, blend almond flour and coconut flour and mix well together. Include preparing soft drinks and salt. Heartbeat to mix. Include dates and heartbeat again until the blend has a similar surface as coarse sand. Mix in apple juice vinegar and eggs and mix well. Heartbeat in the pecans quickly. Pour the hitter on to a smaller than normal portion skillet. Put inside the broiler and heat for 28 to 32 minutes at 350° F. Cool the bread while still in search of gold hours before evacuating. Makes 1 little portion of Walnut Bread.

## Dull Rye Bread

Ingredients:

1 cup almond flour, whitened
½ tsp baking soda

¾ tsp cream of tartar 3 eggs

2 tbsp olive oil

A ¼ cup of water

1 tsp nectar or nectar

1-2 tbsp caraway seeds

Directions:

Blend almond flour, flax, salt, heating soft drink and cream of tartar in an enormous bowl. In a different, littler bowl blend egg, oil, water, and agave. Mix in the dry fixings into wet. Include the caraway seeds and blend well. Let the player represent 1 to 2 minutes for it to thicken. Pour the player to a little, lubed portion container. Prepare for 30-35 minutes at 350° F.

## Paleo Banana Bread

Ingredients:

1 ½ cups bananas (squashed)

1 tbsp nectar

1 tbsp vanilla concentrate

3 eggs

¼ Cup vegetarian shortening

½ tsp ocean salt

2 Cup almond flour, whitened

1 tsp heating soft drink

Guidelines:

Join bananas, nectar, vanilla, eggs, and shortening into the nourishment processor and heartbeat them together. Include the almond flour, heating soft drink, and salt while beating with every expansion. Empty the hitter into a recently lubed portion skillet. Prepare for 50 to an hour at 350°F. Remove from the broiler and cool before expelling from the container.

**Cranberry Loaf Bread**

Ingredients:

¾ C simmered almond spread, at room temperature

3 eggs

2 tbsp olive oil

¼ C arrowroot powder

¼ tsp heating soft drink

almond flour(blanched)

½ cup dried cranberries

olive oil

¼ Cup dried apricots(chopped)

¼ C sesame seeds

1 tsp ocean salt

¼ C sunflower seeds

¼ C pumpkin seeds

¼ cup in addition to

2 tbsp cut almonds.

Guidelines:

Join the eggs, olive oil and almond spread in a huge bowl and mix until smooth utilizing a hand blender In a different medium-size bowl, mix arrowroot powder, preparing soft drink and salt. Mix the wet blend with the arrowroot blend until all around blended. Crease in the cut almonds, dried apricots, sesame seeds, and cranberries.

Oil a portion container with olive oil and powder with almond flour. Move the hitter cautiously into the dish and top uniformly with whatever cut almonds left. Prepare for 40 to 50 minutes at 350° or until a blade embedded into focus tells the truth. Cool the bread for in any event 1 hour while in the skillet before evacuating.

PALEO SOUP RECIPES

**Sopa de Lima**

Ingredients:

4 parts chicken bosom

¼ tsp Chili Powder

4 Cups of Organic Chicken Broth ( you can utilize your very own natively grown juices)

¼ tsp Garlic Powder.

2 pieces Chile Peppers

2 Tomatoes, sliced

4 to 5 Garlic Cloves, stripped and minced.

1 Tbsp Olive Oil

½ of an Onion, chopped

⅓ Cup Lime juice (or you can take the juice from 2 limes)

½ tsp Lime juice

2 Tbsp Cilantro, chopped

1 stripped Avocado, cleaved.

Ocean Salt

Guidelines:

Organize chicken in a preparing dish fixed with oil. Sprinkle the chicken with garlic and stew powder. Spot the heating dish inside the stove preheated to 400 degrees and prepare the Chicken for twenty minutes. Meanwhile, the chicken is preparing in the broiler, set a stockpot over the stove and include the olive oil. Sauté the Garlic, Onion and Serrano peppers together until they are delicate for three minutes. Mix in the Chopped Tomatoes and leave stewing for in any event two minutes more. Include lime juice and chicken stock while mixing once in a while. Alter temperature to low warmth. Expel the chicken from stove following two minutes and cool only enough for you to have the option to deal with it and hack it into little chomp sizes.

Return the slashed chicken pieces to the stockpot, and increment the warmth to carry the blend to bubble. When bubbling, bring down the warmth to the most minimal setting, and put on the top spread. Give it a chance to bubble daintily for an extra 20 minutes on low warmth. Spot the avocado pieces into each serving bowl (not legitimately into soup stock). Put the avocado in each bowl first at that point pour the soup over it. Wrap up by decorating with Cilantro.

## Bacon Soup with Asparagus, Green Peas

Ingredients:

1 bundle asparagus, medium, cut

1/2 white onion, slashed

4 cups of bacon

3 Cup chicken stock (you can utilize vegetable stock as well)

2 cloves garlic, minced

1 C new peas (you can utilize solidified peas however defrost them first)

1/2 cup milk

Directions:

Utilize a wide-bottomed skillet to sear the bacon till they begin to be somewhat fresh. Expel them quickly from the skillet utilizing an opened spoon and set them aside to cool for some time. Disintegrate or Chop the bacon into minor pieces when cool enough. Sauté the onion and garlic utilizing a similar skillet till the onion turns brilliant. Include the peas and asparagus after. Stream in the chicken stock and let it bubble once more. Spread and lower the warmth. Permit to stew for twenty minutes before taking the skillet off the warmth. Utilize a hand-held blender to process the soup until it is smooth. Add flavoring as per taste. Top with bacon bits before serving.

## Hot and Sour Chicken Soup

Ingredients:

2 tbsp Coconut Oil

1 Cup Onion, cut

1/2 cup carrots, diced

1/2 Cup Celery, cut

2 Skinless Chicken Breast-medium diced

6 Cups Chicken Stock

5 Mushrooms, cut

1 tbsp crisp ginger minced

3 cloves garlic

3 tbsp Coconut Aminos

1/2 tsp Honey

3 tbsp White Wine Vinegar

1/2 tsp Sesame Oil

2 tbsp Tapioca Starch broke down in 0.5 cup chicken juices.

6 Eggs, beaten

2 Green Onions Chopped

1/2 Cup Bamboo Shoots meagerly Sliced Salt

Pepper

Hot Chili Oil


Guidelines:


Sauté onions in a substantial pot over medium/high warmth for 3 minutes. Include the carrots and cut onions. Keep on sauté until carrots become delicate. Pour in the chicken stock and hold up till it bubbles. Toss in the mushrooms, ginger, coconut oil, garlic, vinegar, nectar, and sesame oil in a specific order.

Increment the temperature to heat the blend to the point of boiling. Energetically whisk the custard starch with the chicken juices and empty in the custard arrangement into the stockpot with the soup while blending the soup persistently. Enable the soup to bubble once more. Keep on blending until the soup is thick at that point decrease the warmth to medium.

Sprinkle the whisked eggs gradually over the bubbling soup while mixing consistently. Include the green onions, bamboo shoots, pepper, and salt together with a modest quantity of the stew oil. Diminish the warmth to Low this time and let it stew for 5 minutes. Taste the soup. Include more bean stew oil if necessary only a little at any given moment until the taste is zesty enough for you.

**Occasion Bouillabaisse**

Fixings:

1 can diced tomatoes

28 oz crisp cleaved tomatoes

1 onion, medium, slashed

1 medium red ringer pepper

3 to 4 stalks celery, cut and slashed

2 cloves garlic, slashed

½ lb shelled medium shrimps, deveined

¼ lb. swordfish, cleaned and cut in blocks

½ lb. cove scallops

½ tsp cinnamon

1 tsp cumin

cayenne pepper

dark pepper and Salt

2 cups of water

Guidelines:

You ought to have around equivalent volumes of cleaved onions, chile peppers, and celery. Include in any if necessary. Sauté onion, garlic, ringer pepper, and celery, in 3 tablespoon olive oil. Include dark pepper and salt. Include the swordfish 3D shapes and keep on cooking until the vegetables are delicate yet firm. Include the tomatoes, two cups of water, cinnamon and cumin.

Put some of the cayenne pepper as per your preference. Heat it until it boils for five minutes. Include the shrimp and continue boiling the mixture for an additional 4 minutes. Mix in the scallops and keep boiling for one more moment this time. Lessen to low warmth. Close the lid of the container and permit to stew for at the very least 25 minutes and close to 30 minutes. Garnish with crisp parsley sprigs and serve.

PALEO DINNER RECIPES

**Sheep Veggie Stew**

Ingredients :

2 tablespoons olive oil

1 Onion cut

1 Carrot cut

1 Zucchini cut

1 Green pepper cut

1 teaspoon Italian flavoring

1 pound sheep cubed

4 cups of chicken juices

crisp cleaved parsley for serving

Guidelines:

Warmth the oil in an enormous soup pot. Include the vegetables and cook until mellowed. Include the Italian flavoring, and the sheep and cook until sheep are caramelized. Blend in the soup and heat to the point of boiling. Lessen warmth and stew until sheep are delicate. Serve beat with the hacked parsley.

**Cooked Brussels Sprouts with Bacon**

Ingredients

2 pounds Brussels sprouts divided

2 tablespoons olive oil

8 bacon cuts cooked and disintegrated

Ocean salt and new ground pepper to taste

Directions

Put the sprouts in steamer crate or microwave and steam until simply delicate. Evacuate and let cool marginally. Hurl the steamed sprouts with the olive oil and a spot of salt. Lay on a material lined preparing sheet, cut side up. Preheat grill to high warmth and cook until tops are all around caramelized. Hurl with the bacon and serve warm.

## Balsamic Chicken Salad

Ingredients

Chicken

1/2 cup olive oil

1/4 cup Balsamic vinegar

1 teaspoon Dijon mustard

1/2 teaspoon ocean salt

1/4 teaspoon dark pepper

Salad

8 cups hacked Romaine lettuce

2 Large tomatoes quartered

2 cups cooked and hacked green beans

Juice of 2 lemons

1/4 cup olive oil

Directions

Whisk the olive oil, vinegar, and mustard in a little bowl with the salt and pepper. Brush half over the chicken bosoms. Preheat flame broil to medium-high warmth. Barbecue the chicken until cooked through, permit to cool and cut. Prepare the plate of mixed greens in a huge bowl with the lemon juice and olive oil and top with the cut chicken.

**Chicken and Vegetable Bowl**

Ingredients

3 tablespoons olive oil

2 cloves garlic minced

2 Bell peppers any shading, cut

1 Red onion cut

4 cups Spinach slashed

1/2 cup destroyed carrots

2 tablespoons Lemon juice

1/2 cup Chopped crisp parsley

2 cups cooked and destroyed chicken bosom

Sprouts for garnishing

Ocean salt and new ground pepper to taste

Directions

Warmth the oil in an overwhelming bottomed skillet over medium warmth. Include the garlic, peppers, and onion and cook until diminished. Include the spinach and carrots and cook until spinach is withered. Include the parsley and lemon squeeze and mood killer heat. Mix the chicken into the vegetables and serve beat with the sprouts.

**Spring Lamb Stir Fry**

Ingredients:

3 tablespoons Coconut oil

1 pound boneless sheep cubed

2 cloves garlic minced

1 teaspoon crisp ginger

2 Zucchini cut

1 enormous carrot cut

1 teaspoon ground coriander

1 teaspoon ground cumin

Juice of 1 lime

crisp cleaved cilantro

Cauliflower rice for serving

Ocean salt and crisp ground pepper to taste

Guidelines:

Warmth the coconut oil in an enormous skillet. Include the sheep and cook until sautéed. Expel from skillet and include the garlic, ginger, zucchini, and carrots. Cook until mellowed. Include the coriander, cumin, and lime squeeze, and add the sheep back to the container. Keep cooking until sheep is finished. Serve beat with the cilantro and with cauliflower rice.

## Greek Chicken and Veggie Skewers

Ingredients:

Marinade

1/2 cup olive oil

2 lemons, squeezed

1 teaspoon Red wine vinegar

2 tablespoons Chopped crisp parsley

2 tablespoons cleaved new mint

1 teaspoon Oregano

1/2 teaspoon Sea salt

1/2 teaspoon Fresh ground dark pepper

**Sticks**

1.5 pounds boneless chicken cubed

1 half quart Cherry tomatoes

1 Red onion cubed

2 Zucchini cubed

1 half quart Button mushrooms

Instructions:

Mix the marinade ingredients in a container and mix them well. Wire the chicken and greens upon skewers and lay in a shallow dish. Spill the marinade over top. Cool for at least 3 hours, rolling occasionally. When set to cook, take out the skewers from the refrigerator and preheat a gas or charcoal grill to medium-high heat. Grill the skewers until rooster is cooked through and veggies are slightly browned.

**Roasted Vegetables with Bacon**

Ingredients:

4 cuts bacon slashed

1 onion cut

1 pound Brussel sprouts divided

1/2 pound little radishes divided

1/2 head broccoli cut into florets

ocean salt to taste

crisp ground dark pepper to taste

Guidelines:

Heat a big frypan over medium-high flame. Include the bacon and cook until it gets crispy. Expel the bacon from the dish, leaving behind only the fat. Add the onion and cook until mellowed. First, cook the Brussel sprouts and cook them until they are lightly burned and then include the radishes and broccoli in them. Keep cooking them till the veggies are slightly burnt. In the end, add the bacon back to the skillet before you serve the meal.

## Turkey Bowl with Kale and Sweet Potatoes

Ingredients:

3 cups Dinosaur kale (cut into nibble measured pieces)

2 cups Turkey bosom (cooked and cleaved)

1/4 cup dried cranberries

1/4 cup toasted sunflower seeds

1/4 cup olive oil

2 tbsp Cider vinegar

1 tbsp Dijon mustard

2 tbsp real maple syrup

3 strips Cooked bacon (disintegrated)

2 Sweet potatoes (stripped and cubed)

Directions:

Put the sweet potatoes in a pot and spread it with virus water. Heat to the point of boiling and decrease warmth to a stew. Stew for 10 to 15 minutes, until delicate. Channel. Backrub the kale in an enormous bowl for a few minutes, until leaves are delicate and separated. Include the potatoes, cranberries, and sunflower seeds to the bowl. In a different bowl whisk the olive oil, juice vinegar, mustard, maple syrup, and salt and pepper until very much joined. Prepare it with the serving of mixed greens. Include the turkey and bacon before serving.

## Paleo Italian Meatballs and Braised Greens

Ingredients:

2 tbsp olive oil

2 tbsp Italian flavoring

2 cloves garlic (minced)

1/4 cup Almond Flour

1 tsp Paprika

1/2 tsp Sea salt

1/2 lbs ground hamburger

1 Onion (finely slashed)

Greens:

4 cuts bacon (diced)

1 bundle Collard greens (stems evacuated and cleaved)

1 bundle Swiss chard (stems evacuated and cleaved)

1 cup Chicken juices (or water)

2 tsp Apple juice vinegar

Ocean salt and crisp ground pepper

Guidelines:

Preheat broiler to 400 degrees Fahrenheit. Join the hamburger, onion, garlic, almond flour, paprika, and salt in a huge bowl. Utilizing your hands, blend until simply joined, being mindful so as not to over blend. Structure into 2-inch meatballs and lay on a heating sheet. Brush with the olive oil and coat with the Italian flavoring. Heat for 20-30 minutes, until cooked through. To make the greens, cook the bacon an enormous, profound skillet until it begins to darken. Add the greens and mix to coat in the fat. Add the soup or water to cover the greens and go down to low. Give the greens a chance to stew for around 10 minutes over low warmth until greens are delicate. Serve the meatballs over the greens.

**Paleo Buffalo Mushroom Skewers**

Ingredients:

1 pound Button mushrooms

1/2 cup Hot sauce

2 tbsp olive oil

1/2 tsp Sea salt

Directions:

With a paper towel, cautiously clean the mushrooms, yet don't get them wet. Leave entire, yet expel the stems whenever wanted. Whisk the hot sauce, olive oil, and salt in a bowl. Add the mushrooms and hurl to coat. To cook the mushrooms, string them on sticks and lay on a preparing sheet (or on the other hand, you can leave them off the sticks) Bake for 15 minutes in a 375-degree broiler, or flame broils them on a barbecue over medium-high warmth. Serve warm.

PALEO DESSERT RECIPES

**Paleo chocolate chip treats**

Ingredients:

1 egg, marginally beaten

1 teaspoon vanilla concentrate

1/4 cup coconut oil, softened and cooled

1/2 cup coconut sugar

1 cup almond flour

1/4 cup coconut flour

1/2 teaspoon heating soft drink

3 oz 80% dim chocolate, coarsely chopped*

Coarse ocean salt, for sprinkling

Guidelines:

Preheat broiler to 350 degrees Fahrenheit. In a big bowl add beaten egg, softened and cooled coconut oil, coconut sugar, and vanilla concentrate. Next include almond flour, coconut flour, and heating soft drink, blending great to consolidate and frame a batter. Crease in dull chocolate pieces. You may need to utilize your hands to saturate the batter with the goal that it sticks together well. Utilize a treat scoop or huge tablespoon to drop batter onto an ungreased preparing sheet. Tenderly smooth the batter with your hand. Prepare for 11-13 minutes, or until edges are marginally brilliant dark-colored. Sprinkle with coarse ocean salt and permit to cool on the treated sheet for 10 minutes before moving to a wire rack to completing the process of cooling. Makes 12 treats.

**Twofold chocolate hazelnut treats with sea salt**

Ingredients:

2 cups crude hazelnuts

1 teaspoon coconut oil

1/4 teaspoon salt

2/3 cup coconut sugar

1/2 teaspoon vanilla concentrate

1 egg

1 egg yolk

1/2 cup great quality unsweetened cocoa powder

1 teaspoon baking soda

3 oz your preferred dull chocolate bar, slashed (in any event 72%, with no soy)

**Coarse ocean salt, for sprinkling**

Directions:

Preheat stove to 350 degrees F. Equally spread hazelnuts onto an enormous preparing sheet. Toast the hazelnuts in the stove for 8-10 minutes. Expel from the stove and let cool for 5-10 minutes. Keep heat in the stove. Move hazelnuts to the bowl of a nourishment processor and procedure for 10-15 minutes or until it transforms into a hazelnut spread; you'll likely need to scratch down the sides now and again. We need this to be velvety so try to get it that way. When it begins to get velvety, include a teaspoon of coconut oil and the salt and procedure again for one more moment or two. Presently let the nut margarine sit for 5-10 minutes until it chills off a bit. This is significant so remember to do it! Else you'll finish up with a cooked egg. Include the coconut sugar, vanilla, egg, and additional egg yolk. Procedure again until all-around joined and a battery starts to shape. Next include cocoa powder and baking soda, and procedure once more. The mixture may turn into an enormous ball, so if that happens simply move the batter to a medium bowl and utilize a wooden spoon to blend everything until all-around joined. Next mix in slashed chocolate. Structure batter into 1/2 inch balls, place on treat sheet and level the mixture with the palm of your hand. I like to level mine quite dainty. Prepare for 8-10 minutes at that point expel from broiler and sprinkle with ocean salt. Enable treats to cool on the treated sheet for a couple of minutes before moving to a wire rack to cool totally.

Makes around 18 treats

## Paleo No-Bake Cookie Dough Truffles

Ingredients:

½ tablespoon flaxseed seed

1 tablespoon unsweetened almond milk

2 tablespoons softened coconut oil

3 tablespoons coconut sugar

1 teaspoon vanilla concentrate

½ cup pressed almond flour

2 tablespoons coconut flour

⅛ teaspoon salt

1½ tablespoon dim chocolate chips, dairy-free whenever wanted

**For the chocolate covering:**

⅓ cup dim chocolate chips, dairy-free whenever wanted

1 teaspoon coconut oil

Directions:

In a medium bowl combine flaxseed dinner, almond milk, liquefied coconut oil, vanilla, and coconut sugar. In a little bowl combine almond flour, coconut flour, and salt. Gradually add the flour blend to the wet fixings. Blend well until a treat mixture consistency shapes. Crease chocolate chips into the treat mixture. Fold treat mixture into 1 tablespoon estimated balls, place on material lined preparing sheet and stop for 10 minutes. Following 10 minutes, soften the chocolate chips and coconut oil in a little pan over exceptionally low warmth, blending much of the time. You can likewise microwave the chocolate in a little microwave-safe bowl in 20-second augmentations until softened. Rapidly utilize a fork to plunge every treat batter ball into the chocolate, trying to coat uniformly. Move back to material fixed preparing sheet and sprinkle with a little coarse ocean salt whenever wanted. Promptly spot heating sheet back in cooler for 20 minutes. Makes 8 treat mixture chomps. Keep in cooler until prepared to eat.

**Paleo Banana Zucchini Muffins**

Ingredients:

1 cup destroyed zucchini (from 1 medium zucchini)

1/2 cup squashed banana (from 1 medium banana)

3/4 cup cashew margarine

1/4 cup unadulterated maple syrup

2 eggs

1 teaspoon vanilla concentrate

1/2 cup coconut flour

1 teaspoon heating soft drink

1/4 teaspoon salt

Guidelines:

Preheat broiler to 350 degrees F. Line a biscuit tin with 10 biscuit liners. You're just making 10 biscuits, so forget two liners. Press destroyed zucchini of overabundance dampness with a paper towel. In a huge bowl, include zucchini, banana, cashew spread, maple syrup, eggs, and vanilla. Blend until smooth and all-around consolidated. Next add the dry fixings to the wet fixings: coconut flour, heating soft drink, and salt. Blend until consolidated. Separation player equitably between 10 biscuit cups. Prepare for 22-27 minute or until toothpick confesses all and the highest points of the biscuits are simply marginally brilliant dark-colored. Makes 10 biscuits.

# CHAPTER 13

## CONCLUSION AND PROPOSAL

I assume that this fashion is worth giving an attempt to seeing for yourself if you'll be able to comply with this lifestyle or not.

One amongst the main issue that this fashion has extremely done is that it's helped heaps of individuals with their weight and health connected problems particularly and folks usually have seen their bodies remodeling from corpulent to slim and lean and it's one of the good virtues of the Paleo diet and one of the main attraction of this diet style and if paleo diet has worked for those people then it can even work for you,but it all depends on you whether or not you would like to give it an attempt or not. however, with thereupon they are also are other things to stay in mind whereas considering beginning the Paleo diet:

What level of processed food is suitable to you, by that term I mean the food that's changed in a way like canned goods, etc. you've got to see what level of processed food you're able to incorporate in your diet plan. there's no proper way to certify what Paleo diet is, therefore, this generally gets confusing for folks to outline what Paleo is, therefore, you would like to try and do your analysis furthermore to seek out what you actually ascertain Paleo diet to be for yourself and incorporate that diet set up in your lifestyle.

You would have to rule out the skepticism within the validity of Paleo and therefore to try and do that you just got to verify what folks consider Paleo collectively to rule out ambiguity.


The end to all the discussion above is that the message is unbelievably obvious which is that the modern western eating routine that comprises of high  and high carb nourishments isn't getting the opportunity to work for your well being and shape inside the long run and you would need to change over back to the sustenances that are suitable for the figure along these lines you have to ask yourself instructed as far as Paleo diet and join in your life though for a short amount of your opportunity to look at anyway the outcomes commencement to be and on the off chance that get happy with the consequence of this eating regimen set up, at that point voila you've discovered the enchantment key to great well being and readiness for an amazing remainder.

Along these lines, at last, all I ask of you is to give this eating regimen plan a month's time and that I am very positive that in the event that you pursue this eating regimen plan for a month's time you'll probably not be coming back to the high sugar, high sodium diet that we are accustomed to having by and by. So I wish you a glad Paleo and good luck for what's to come.